INTENSIVE DIABETES MANAGEMENT

SIXTH EDITION

Edited by
Howard Wolpert, MD

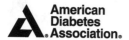

**American
Diabetes
Association.**

Director, Book Publishing, Abe Ogden; *Managing Editor,* Rebekah Renshaw; *Acquisitions Editor,* Victor Van Beuren; *Production Manager and Composition,* Melissa Sprott; *Cover Design,* Jody Billert; *Printer,* Data Reproductions Corp.

Printed in the United States of America
1 3 5 7 9 10 8 6 4 2

The suggestions and information contained in this publication are generally consistent with the *Standards of Medical Care in Diabetes* and other policies of the American Diabetes Association, but they do not represent the policy or position of the Association or any of its boards or committees. Reasonable steps have been taken to ensure the accuracy of the information presented. However, the American Diabetes Association cannot ensure the safety or efficacy of any product or service described in this publication. Individuals are advised to consult a physician or other appropriate health care professional before undertaking any diet or exercise program or taking any medication referred to in this publication. Professionals must use and apply their own professional judgment, experience, and training and should not rely solely on the information contained in this publication before prescribing any diet, exercise, or medication. The American Diabetes Association—its officers, directors, employees, volunteers, and members—assumes no responsibility or liability for personal or other injury, loss, or damage that may result from the suggestions or information in this publication.

∞ The paper in this publication meets the requirements of the ANSI Standard Z39.48-1992 (permanence of paper).

ADA titles may be purchased for business or promotional use or for special sales. To purchase more than 50 copies of this book at a discount, or for custom editions of this book with your logo, contact the American Diabetes Association at the address below, at booksales@diabetes.org, or by calling 703-299-2046.

American Diabetes Association
1701 North Beauregard Street
Alexandria, Virginia 22311

DOI: 10.2337/9781580406321

Library of Congress Cataloging-in-Publication Data
Names: Wolpert, Howard, 1958- , editor. | American Diabetes Association, issuing body.
Title: Intensive diabetes management / [edited by] Howard Wolpert.
Description: 6th edition. | Alexandria : American Diabetes Association, [2016] | Includes bibliographical references and index.
Identifiers: LCCN 2016014046 | ISBN 9781580406321 (alk. paper)
Subjects: | MESH: Diabetes Mellitus--therapy | Diet, Diabetic | Insulin--administration & dosage | Patient Education as Topic | Self Care--methods
Classification: LCC RC660 | NLM WK 815 | DDC 616.4/62--dc23
LC record available at http://lccn.loc.gov/2016014046

Contents

Contributors to the Sixth Edition

Kirstine Bell, RD, CDE, PhD
Research Fellow, University of Sydney,
  Australia.

Ann Goebel-Fabbri, PhD
Past Senior Psychologist,
  Joslin Diabetes Center
Assistant Professor of Psychiatry,
  Harvard Medical School

Marilyn Ritholz, PhD
Senior Psychologist,
  Joslin Diabetes Center
Assistant Professor of Psychiatry,
  Harvard Medical School

Jo-Anne Rizzotto, MEd, RD, LDN, CDE
Director, Educational Services,
  Joslin Diabetes Center

Emmy Suhl, MS, RD, CDE, LD
Senior Nutritionist,
  Joslin Diabetes Center

Elena Toschi, MD
Staff Physician,
  Joslin Diabetes Center
Instructor in Medicine,
  Harvard Medical School

Howard Wolpert, MD
Senior Physician,
  Joslin Diabetes Center/Beth Israel
  Deaconess Medical Center
Associate Professor of Medicine,
  Harvard Medical School

Rationale for and Physiological Basis of Intensive Diabetes Management

DOI: 10.2337/9781580406321.01

Highlights
Rationale for and
Physiological Basis of
Intensive Diabetes Management

- Technological and pharmacological innovations have made it possible for individuals with diabetes to achieve near-normal glycemic control.

- The goal of intensive diabetes management is to achieve near-normal glycemia. This mode of treatment has been shown in large prospective randomized studies as the preferred approach for many patients with diabetes to delay the onset and progression of albuminuria in patients with both type 1 and type 2 diabetes.

- Glycemic control that approaches the nondiabetic state postpones or slows the progression of the retinal, renal, and neurological complications of diabetes.

- Glycemic control that approaches the nondiabetic state lowers risk factors that promote macrovascular disease (e.g., plasminogen activator inhibitor–1 levels; platelet aggregation; small, dense low-density lipoprotein cholesterol particles).

- Intensive diabetes management is successful when insulin is delivered and adjusted in amounts required by changes in nutritional intake (e.g., amounts of carbohydrate, protein, fat), physical activity, and associated internal and external stresses. Successful management of these issues will approximate normal fuel metabolism.

- Self-monitoring of blood glucose is performed to guide adjustments in insulin dosage in relation to food consumption and, especially, carbohydrate intake, activity variation, and ambient blood glucose levels to ideally achieve

  • a relatively constant, low plasma-free insulin level during fasting (postabsorptive state);

  • a rapid increase in plasma-free insulin after meals, in an amount appropriate to the amount of food (primarily carbohydrate) eaten; and

  • a decrease in plasma-free insulin levels especially during and after prolonged, strenuous exercise or when food intake is delayed.

Rationale for and Physiological Basis of Intensive Diabetes Management

Diabetes management aims to achieve near-normal glycemic control to prevent or ameliorate diabetes complications. The effectiveness of glycemic control in reducing the risk of microvascular and neuropathic complications is well established. Technical advances such as self-monitoring of blood glucose (SMBG), the measurement of glycated hemoglobin A_{1c}, continuous glucose monitoring (CGM), insulin analogs, and the availability of technically advanced smart insulin pumps have provided the tools for successful intensive diabetes management.

Studies in type 1 diabetes (T1D), type 2 diabetes (T2D), and in pregnant women with diabetes have shown benefits sufficient to prompt a consensus on intensive glycemic control as a standard of care. The landmark Diabetes Control and Complications Trial (DCCT) showed that glycemic control (achieving mean A1C of 7.1%) postpones, prevents, or slows the progression of retinal, renal, and neurological complications. Follow-up of the DCCT cohort in the Epidemiology of Diabetes Interventions and Complications (EDIC) study has shown persistence of the beneficial effects in the intensively treated subjects even though their glycemic control during follow-up has been equivalent to that of subjects in the conventional treatment arm of the DCCT. Glucose lowering in the intensive treatment arm also was associated with long-term benefit with regard to cardiovascular complications. Intensive treatment, therefore, should be started as soon as is safely possible after the onset of T1D and maintained thereafter aiming for a practicable target A1C level of ≤7.0% provided that this can be achieved safely and without frequent and severe hypoglycemia.

In T2D, the UK Prospective Diabetes Study (UKPDS) in patients with new-onset T2D and the Kumamoto Study in Japan, similarly, demonstrated significant reductions in microvascular and neuropathic complications with intensive therapy. The majority of patients with diabetes succumb to heart attack, stroke, or their consequences. The potential of intensive glycemic control to reduce cardiovascular disease in T2D is supported by epidemiological studies and a meta-analysis. Three randomized controlled trials, the Action to Control Cardiovascular Risk in Diabetes [ACCORD], Action in Diabetes and Vascular Disease: Preterax and Diamicron Modified Release Controlled Evaluation [ADVANCE], and Veterans Affairs Diabetes Trial [VADT]), however, showed that targeting near-normal A1C in high-risk patients with T2D did not have a beneficial effect on cardiovascular disease. Indeed, a treatment strategy designed to lower blood glucose to near-normal levels in the ACCORD trial was associated with increased mortality.

DOI: 10.2337/9781580406321.01

Although glucose management clearly is important, aggressive management of blood pressure and lipids, smoking cessation, and antiplatelet therapy are critically important aspects of care, can dramatically reduce the rate of cardiovascular events, and must be a major focus of therapy.

Patients with T1D across the age spectrum as well as many patients with T2D increasingly are adopting intensive management strategies. Indeed, some elderly patients with longstanding T2D experience control resembling that of an insulin-deficient patient, having wide swings of blood glucose, and sensitivity to timing or small differences of insulin dose, such that intensive management may be especially appropriate in their care. Patients with long life expectancy, without advanced diabetes complications, or without hypoglycemia unawareness may benefit from this management strategy.

INTENSIVE DIABETES MANAGEMENT

Intensive diabetes management is a mode of treatment in which the goal is euglycemia or near-normal glycemia. Achieving this goal involves the integration of several diabetes treatment components into the individual's lifestyle. These components may include

- an individualized medication regimen;
- frequent blood glucose monitoring;
- CGM;
- the use of pre- and postprandial SMBG data, blood glucose patterns, and trends to meet individually defined treatment goals;
- active adjustment of medication, food, or activity based on blood glucose measurements;
- active use of carbohydrate counting as a strategy to match food with insulin;
- ongoing interaction between the individual with diabetes and the health-care team;
- assessment, including
  - education,
  - medical care and treatment,
  - emotional and psychological support, and
  - frequent objective assessment of glycemic control (A1C measurement).

In addition, a thorough understanding of diabetes and its management by all professional personnel involved in the daily care of diabetes is crucial.

Most patients with T1D will require multiple daily insulin injections or an insulin pump to achieve the goals of treatment. For patients with T2D, successful intensified therapy (with goals similar to those in T1D) may be possible with lifestyle interventions (regular physical exercise and careful medical nutrition therapy to lose weight). In patients with T2D with greater degrees of insulin deficiency, oral glucose-lowering medications (biguanides, sulfonylureas, thiazolidinediones, glinides, α-glucosidase inhibitors, dipeptidyl peptidase-IV inhibitors, sodium glucose cotransporter inhibitors) given singly or in combination, noninsulin injectable glucose-lowering medications (glucagon-like peptide-1 analogs, amylin analogs), or insulin are needed to achieve near-normal glycemia. The goals of therapy may be modified in some patients because of age, comorbid states, ability to adhere to a schedule of regular follow-up assessments, or other individual clinical situations that make the risks of intensified diabetes management greater than the benefits. The balance between risk and benefit may be more delicate in the child without appropriate family support or in the elderly patient.

PHYSIOLOGICAL BASIS OF INTENSIVE MANAGEMENT METHODS

Intensive diabetes management attempts to normalize fuel metabolism by delivering insulin or oral diabetes medications to approximate normal physiology. Although the goal of completely normal physiology cannot be achieved with available methods, it is possible to improve glycemic control enough to have a dramatic impact on the risk of chronic complications.

NORMAL FUEL METABOLISM

Fuel metabolism is regulated by a complex system involving

- multiple tissues and organs;
- intracellular enzyme systems to use nutrient fuels; and
- hormones and other regulatory factors to
  - distribute ingested nutrients to organs and tissues according to the needs for mechanical or chemical work and tissue growth or renewal,
  - provide storage of excess nutrients as glycogen and fat, and
  - allow release of energy from storage depots as needed during periods of fasting or exercise.

Carbohydrate Metabolism

Glucose is a major energy source for muscles and the brain. The brain is nearly totally dependent on glucose, whereas muscles also use fat and ketone bodies for fuel. The two main sources of circulating glucose are hepatic glucose production and ingested carbohydrate. After absorption of a meal is complete, glucose production by the liver supplies all the glucose needed for tissues such as the brain that do not store glucose. This is referred to as *basal glucose production* and is generally ~2 mg/kg body wt/min in adults. With increasing duration of a fast, as hepatic glycogen stores are exhausted, the relative contribution of gluconeogenesis to basal glucose production increases; however, normally ~50% of basal glucose production is from glycogenolysis; the rest is from gluconeogenesis.

Ingested carbohydrate is hydrolyzed into component glucose during intestinal digestion and monosaccharides are absorbed, producing a postprandial increase in blood glucose level that peaks 60–120 min after the meal. The magnitude and rate of increase in blood glucose are determined by many factors, including the size of the meal, its carbohydrate content, the physical state of the food (e.g., solid, liquid, cooked, raw), the presence of other nutrients (e.g., fat and fiber, which slow digestion), the amount of insulin, and the individual's sensitivity to insulin. The rate of gastric emptying also modulates postprandial blood glucose levels. These factors, in addition to the glycemic index and amount of ingested carbohydrate, have significant effects on glycemia.

Glucose is either oxidized for energy or stored as glycogen or fat. After ingestion of oral carbohydrate, 60–70% is stored, mostly as glycogen; the remainder is oxidized for immediate energy needs.

Protein Metabolism

Ingested protein is absorbed as amino acids, which may be used in three ways:

1. synthesis of new protein
2. oxidation to provide energy
3. conversion to glucose (gluconeogenesis)

During fasting, proteolysis and conversion of gluconeogenic amino acids to glucose prevent hypoglycemia. Alanine is the major amino acid substrate for hepatic gluconeogenesis; glutamine is the major amino acid substrate for renal gluconeogenesis. Branched-chain amino acids may be used for protein synthesis or oxidized for energy. They are the major donors of amino groups for synthesis of alanine, which can be readily converted to glucose.

Fat Metabolism

Fat is the major form of stored energy. Fat stored as triglyceride is converted to free fatty acids and glycerol by lipolysis. Free fatty acids from adipose tissue may be transported to muscle for oxidation. Oxidation of free fatty acids in the liver produces the ketone bodies acetoacetate and β-hydroxybutyrate (referred to as *ketogenesis*). Synthesis of ketone bodies is, therefore, a stage in fat oxidation; they can be oxidized in extrahepatic tissues to produce energy. Much of the ingested fat in a meal is efficiently stored in adipose tissue or muscle. Normally, only a small fraction of a glucose load is taken up by fat cells. In states of chronic excess nutrition, however, ingested fat is not oxidized and excess nutrients (glucose) are converted to fat and stored in adipose tissue. Elevated circulating free fatty acids from ingested fat or lipolysis blunt peripheral insulin action and slow the postabsorptive decrease in blood glucose.

REGULATION OF FUEL METABOLISM

Fuel metabolism is regulated by several hormones. The central nervous system (CNS) has an important role in this regulation, either through hormones or in other ways that are incompletely understood. The major hormones and their effects are summarized in Table 1.1 and discussed in more detail later in this chapter.

Insulin

Insulin is the major hypoglycemic hormone. It acts on liver, fat, and skeletal muscle to increase glucose uptake, oxidation, and storage and to decrease glucose production. Insulin also inhibits lipolysis and thereby limits the availability of fatty acids for oxidation and limits ketogenesis.

Table 1.1—Regulation of Fuel Metabolism by Hormones

	Insulin	Glucagon	Catecholamine	Cortisol	Growth Hormone
Glucose uptake	+	0	–	–	–
Gluconeogenesis	–	+	+	+	+
Glycogenolysis	–	+	+	+	+
Lipolysis	–	+	+	+	+
Ketogenesis	–	+	+	+	+

+, increases; –, decreases; 0, no effect.

Insulin is secreted in two major patterns—basal and prandial. Basal secretion produces relatively constant, low plasma insulin levels that restrain lipolysis and glucose production. Abnormally low levels of basal insulin secretion result in markedly increased glucose production, lipolysis, and ketogenesis, causing hyperglycemia, hyper-fatty acidemia, and ketosis. During exercise, skeletal muscle and other tissues require access to stored energy. Insulin secretion decreases to make stored energy available by allowing increased glucose production and lipolysis to occur. The blood glucose level is the dominant stimulus for insulin secretion. β-cells of the pancreatic islet constantly monitor glucose levels so that insulin secretion is closely linked to changes in glycemia. Even small increases in blood glucose concentrations normally cause an increase in insulin secretion. Prandial insulin secretion rapidly increases to a level many times greater than basal levels. Higher postprandial insulin levels completely suppress hepatic glucose production and lipolysis and stimulate uptake of ingested glucose by insulin-sensitive tissues.

Counterregulatory Hormones

Glucagon, catecholamines (epinephrine and norepinephrine), cortisol, and growth hormone are termed *counterregulatory hormones* because their actions are opposite to those of insulin. Together with insulin, they regulate metabolism under widely varying conditions. These hormones often are referred to as *stress hormones* because their levels in the circulation increase in response to stress. It has been suggested that this response is designed to provide the extra energy that may be needed to cope with stress. The concept of hypoglycemia-associated autonomic failure (HAAF) in diabetes posits that recent antecedent iatrogenic hypoglycemia causes both defective glucose counterregulation (by reducing the epinephrine response to falling glucose levels in the setting of an absent glucagon response) and hypoglycemia unawareness (by reducing the autonomic and the resulting neurogenic symptom responses) and thus a vicious cycle of recurrent hypoglycemia. Perhaps the most compelling support of HAAF is the finding that as few as 2–3 weeks of avoidance of hypoglycemia reverses hypoglycemia unawareness and improves the reduced epinephrine component of defective glucose counterregulation in most affected individuals.

Glucagon. Glucagon is the first line of defense against hypoglycemia in people who do not have diabetes. When blood glucose levels fall, the plasma glucagon concentration rapidly increases, and glucagon potently and rapidly stimulates hepatic glucose production by increasing glycogenolysis and gluconeogenesis. In T1D, despite the loss of β-cell function, glucagon secretion by the pancreatic α-cells persists. Glucagon secretion can promote hepatic glucogenesis inappropriate to ambient glucose elevations, which in part is responsible for triggering fasting hyperglycemia and mediating the rise of glucose that occurs despite fasting or emesis when insulin levels are insufficient. Conversely, appropriate glucagon responsiveness to hypoglycemia is lost among many people with long-standing diabetes, especially if their diabetes has been tightly controlled, resulting in the loss of this important defense mechanism against hypoglycemia.

Catecholamines. Catecholamines are produced at times of stress (fight or flight) and also stimulate the release of stored energy. Epinephrine stimulates glucose production and limits glucose utilization in insulin-sensitive tissues, such as skeletal muscle. Catecholamines are the major defense against hypoglycemia in patients with T1D who have lost their glucagon response to hypoglycemia. Hypoglycemia unawareness and sluggish recovery from hypoglycemia may occur when this defense is defective. Patients with hypoglycemia unawareness are at considerably increased risk for severe and prolonged hypoglycemia, and should embark on intensified glucose control only with great caution after a period of hypoglycemia avoidance and restoration of catecholamine responsiveness.

Cortisol. Secretion of the hormone cortisol also increases at times of stress. Its major effect is to stimulate gluconeogenesis; however, the onset of this effect is much slower than that of glucagon. The hyperglycemic response to cortisol is delayed for several hours. Consequently, cortisol is not effective in protecting against acute hypoglycemia. Cortisol also limits glucose utilization in several tissues including skeletal muscle.

Growth hormone. Growth hormone also has slow effects on glucose metabolism. A major surge of growth hormone secretion occurs during sleep and is responsible for an increase in insulin resistance in the early morning, termed the *dawn phenomenon.* Normally, a slight increase in insulin secretion compensates for the effects of nocturnal growth hormone secretion, but in diabetes, the result may be morning hyperglycemia.

IMPLICATIONS FOR THERAPY

The most effective treatment regimens for diabetes attempt to replicate normal physiology. Important elements of treatment include

- a relatively constant low blood insulin level during fasting,
- a rapid increase in blood insulin levels with meals, in an amount appropriate to the quantity and macronutrient content of food eaten,
- a decrease in insulin levels with vigorous and especially prolonged exercise or prolonged fasting, and
- frequent blood glucose measurements and CGM to guide adjustments in insulin dose and other components of the regimen.

Even the most complicated insulin regimen cannot account for all the conditions that influence blood glucose levels. Indeed, variable absorption of insulin from its subcutaneous injection site is one important factor contributing to blood glucose variation. Therefore, even the best methods currently available do not produce "perfect control." Patients with diabetes may adhere to every aspect of management and still experience unexplained blood glucose variations. These patients should be counseled to expect some variability in blood glucose levels that may be difficult or impossible to account for. Nonetheless, meticulous attention to many small details greatly improves the control that can be achieved.

BIBLIOGRAPHY

Ahern J, Boland E, Doane R, Ahern J, Rose P, Vincent M, Tamborlane WV. Insulin pump therapy in pediatrics: a therapeutic alternative to safely lower HbA1c levels across all age groups. *Pediatr Diabetes* 2002;3:10–15

American Diabetes Association. Standards of medical care in diabetes–2016. *Diabetes Care* 2016;39(Suppl. 1):S1–S111

Cryer PE. Diverse causes of hypoglycemia-associated autonomic failure in diabetes. *N Engl J Med* 2004;350:2272-2279.

Cryer PE. Hypoglycemia-associated autonomic failure in diabetes. *Am J Physiol Endocrinol Metab* 2001;281(6):E1115–E1121

Diabetes Control and Complications Trial (DCCT) Research Group. The effect of intensive treatment of diabetes on the development and progression of long-term complications in insulin-dependent diabetes mellitus. *N Engl J Med* 1993;329:977–986

Diabetes Control and Complications Trial (DCCT) Research Group. Hypoglycemia in the Diabetes Control and Complications Trial. *Diabetes* 1997;46:271–286

Diabetes Control and Complications Trial/Epidemiology of Diabetes Interventions and Complications Research Group. Effect of intensive therapy on the microvascular complications of type 1 diabetes mellitus. *JAMA* 2002;287:2563–2569

Diabetes Control and Complications Trial/Epidemiology of Diabetes Interventions and Complications Research Group. Sustained effect of intensive treatment of type 1 diabetes mellitus on development and progression of diabetic nephropathy: the Epidemiology of Diabetes Interventions and Complications (EDIC) study. *JAMA* 2003;22:290:2159–2167

Gaede P, Vedel P, Larsen N, Jensen GV, Parving HH, Pedersen O. Multifactorial intervention and cardiovascular disease in patients with type 2 diabetes. *N Engl J Med* 2003;348:383–393

Gray A, Raikou M, McGuire A, Fenn P, Stevens R, Cull C, Stratto I, Adler A, Holman R, Turner R. Cost effectiveness of an intensive blood glucose control policy in patients with type 2 diabetes: economic analysis alongside a randomised controlled trial (UKPDS 41): UK Prospective Diabetes Study Group. *BMJ* 2000;320:1373–1378

Hirsch IB. Insulin analogues. *N Engl J Med* 2005;352:174–183

Holman RR, Paul SK, Bethel MA, Matthews DR, Neil HA. 10-year follow-up of intensive glucose control in type 2 diabetes. *N Engl J Med* 2008;359: 1577-1589

Juvenile Diabetes Research Foundation Continuous Glucose Monitoring Study Group. Continuous glucose monitoring and intensive treatment of type 1 diabetes. *N Engl J Med* 2008;359:1464–1476

Kitzmiller JL, Block JM, Brown FL, Catalano PM, Conway DL, Coustan DR, et al. Managing preexisting diabetes for pregnancy: summary of evidence and consensus recommendations for care. *Diabetes Care* 2008;31:1060–1079

Lepore G, Dodesini AR, Nosari I, Trevisan R. Both continuous subcutaneous insulin infusion and a multiple daily insulin injection regimen with glargine as basal insulin are equally better than traditional multiple daily insulin injection treatment. *Diabetes Care* 2003;26:1321–1322

Linkeschova R, Raoul M, Bott U, Berger M, Spraul M. Less severe hypoglycaemia, better metabolic control, and improved quality of life in type 1 diabetes mellitus with continuous subcutaneous insulin infusion (CSII) therapy: an observational study of 100 consecutive patients followed for a mean of 2 years. *Diabet Med* 2002;19:746–751

Martin CL, Albers J, Herman WH, Cleary P, Waberski B, Greene DA, Stevens MJ, Feldman EL. Neuropathy among the Diabetes Control and Complications Trial cohort 8 years after trial completion. *Diabetes Care* 2006;29:340–344

Nathan DM, Cleary PA, Backlund JY, Genuth SM, Lachin JM, Orchard TJ, Raskin P, Zinman B. Intensive diabetes treatment and cardiovascular disease in patients with type 1 diabetes. *N Engl J Med* 2005;353:2643–2653

Nathan DM, Lachin J, Cleary P, Orchard T, Brillon DJ, Backlund JY, O'Leary DH, Genuth SM. Intensive diabetes therapy and carotid intima-media thickness in type 1 diabetes mellitus. *N Engl J Med* 2003;348:2294–2303

Nathan DM, Zinman B, Cleary PA, Backlund JY, Genuth S, Miller R, et al. Modern-day clinical course of type 1 diabetes mellitus after 30 years' duration: the Diabetes Control and Complications Trial/Epidemiology of Diabetes Interventions and Complications and Pittsburgh Epidemiology of Diabetes Complication Experience (1983–2005). *Arch Intern Med* 2009;27;169:1307–1316

Skyler JS, Bergenstal R, Bonow RO, Buse J, Deedwania P, Gale EAM, Howard BV, Kirkman MS, Kosiborod M, Reaven P, Sherwin R. Intensive glycemic control and the prevention of cardiovascular events: implications of the ACCORD, ADVANCE, and VA diabetes trials: a position statement of the American Diabetes Association and a scientific statement of the American College of Cardiology Foundation and the American Heart Association. *Diabetes Care* 2009;32:187–192

Storlien LH, Baur LA, Kriketos AD, Pan DA, Cooney GJ, Jenkins AB, Calvert GD, Campbell LV. Dietary fats and insulin action. *Diabetologia* 1996;39:621–631

Stratton IM, Adler AI, Neil HA, Matthews DR, Mansley SE, Cull CA, Hadden D, Turner RC, Holman RR. Association of glycemia with macrovascular and microvascular complications of type 2 diabetes (UKPDS 35): prospective observational study. *BMJ* 2000;321:405–412

White NH, Clearly PA, Dahms W, Goldstein D, Malone J, Tamborlane WV. Beneficial effects of intensive therapy of diabetes during adolescence: outcomes after the conclusion of the Diabetes Control and Complications Trial (DCCT). *J Pediatr* 2001;139:804–812

The Team Approach

DOI: 10.2337/9781580406321.02

Highlights
The Team Approach

- Multidisciplinary team management is an effective and efficient approach to providing multidimensional care and support for optimal diabetes treatment.
- Multidisciplinary team management provides the patient with
  - medical diagnosis and treatment;
  - focused diabetes self-management education;
  - medical nutrition therapy and nutrition management assistance; and
  - psychosocial evaluation and support.
- Team management necessitates
  - identification of a shared philosophy of care and common treatment goals;
  - collaborative decision making and mutual respect;
  - open and ongoing communication; and
  - active involvement by all team members.
- The treatment plan must be individualized and incorporate
  - medical priorities and concerns; and
  - the patient's abilities, motivation, readiness, and resources.
- Active teamwork requires the patient to
  - become involved in daily self-care;
  - acquire the skills necessary to make reasoned decisions;
  - implement the necessary treatment interventions;
  - maintain frequent, open, and honest communication with health-care providers; and
  - advocate for personal self-care needs.
- Health-care provider responsibilities are to
  - develop rapport and trust through nonjudgmental communication;
  - establish treatment goals collaboratively;
  - inform and educate;
  - negotiate needed lifestyle changes; and
  - facilitate achievement of knowledgeable independence in self-care.

- Effective team communication requires
  - clear role expectations;
  - flexible professional boundaries;
  - shared responsibility;
  - an open approach to management interventions; and
  - mutual respect among team members.
- Patients should hear the same message from team members to avoid confusion and undermining of treatment.

The Team Approach

The American Diabetes Association (ADA) supports the position that intensive diabetes management should be considered for most patients with diabetes. Like that of many other chronic diseases, management of diabetes requires that lifestyle issues be addressed if the interventions are to be accepted and successfully integrated. Few disorders, however, demand such a high level of daily attention to behavioral issues and choices. Although most health-care providers recognize the existence of these issues, objective analysis of current diabetes health-care practices reveals a significant and continued discrepancy between this knowledge and actual practice patterns. The message that *glycemic control matters* must be translated into individually defined health-care choices and treatment decisions.

Multidisciplinary team management has become the gold standard for providing the multidimensional care and support that diabetes demands. This approach emphasizes focused diabetes education, nutrition management, interventions that enhance physical fitness, and psychosocial support, all of which complement the traditional medical model that includes diagnosis and treatment. Lack of time and multidimensional expertise are significant constraints to providing this quality of care. In the presence of irrefutable data that intensive diabetes management is beneficial, appropriate care can no longer be expected to occur in the context of two to four 10-minute medical management visits per year. In stark contrast, the intensive management group of the Diabetes Control and Complications Trial (DCCT) received monthly appointments with the study health-care team and even more frequent phone calls from staff who reviewed blood glucose patterns and adjusted insulin regimens accordingly. The team also provided valuable encouragement and support. This level of intervention is not feasible within the bounds of current health-care models; however, providing multidisciplinary care may be the best available approximation and compromise.

Management of diabetes necessitates active involvement, open communication, and mutual understanding by both the patient and the health-care team (see Table 2.1). Ongoing diabetes care can be most effectively carried out in the context of this trusting relationship.

INTEGRATED DIABETES MANAGEMENT TEAM

The individual with diabetes is the central member of the diabetes team and is guided in self-care practices and interventions by the team's professional members. The patient's self-management efforts can be further supported by individu-

Table 2.1—Factors That Influence Team Function

- Common goals and objectives
- Role expectations of each team member, *including* the patient
- Decision-making and communication process
- Leadership style

als who play important roles in the patient's day-to-day life, such as spouses, significant others, parents, children, teachers, friends, and coworkers. The patient must be engaged to make the commitment to self-care and be an active participant in his or her health care or, progress will be limited. Active participation includes

- demonstrating commitment to work at intensive treatment;
- acquiring the necessary skills to manage treatment changes;
- making ongoing decisions regarding daily management;
- identifying and addressing factors affecting the treatment plan; and
- maintaining frequent, open, and honest communication with the health-care team.

Health-care providers have the responsibility to inform and educate the patient about available treatment options, work with the patient to establish treatment goals, and then negotiate and promote needed lifestyle changes (see Table 2.2). The goal of intervention is to facilitate knowledgeable and independent self-care based on the individual's abilities. Ongoing communication (problem solving, feedback, and support) guides the patient's efforts. Patient education programs should incorporate

- technical skills training,
- guidelines for individualized dietary and physical activity approaches,
- problem-solving techniques,
- guidance regarding risk management and management of diabetes comorbidities, and
- identification of interpersonal and practical supports that will enable patients to intensify their care regimen and maintain their progress.

Table 2.2—Health-Care Provider Responsibilities

- Utilize open and nonjudgmental communication
- Understand aspects of the patient's life outside of diabetes, especially those that might affect diabetes management
- Know the current American Diabetes Association's (ADA's) Clinical Practice Recommendations and their scientific and clinical basis
- Use ADA's Clinical Practice Recommendations to define and evaluate diabetes care delivery and practices
- Implement an effective treatment plan through ongoing patient education and communication
- Foster appropriate independence in self-care practices
- Provide ongoing feedback and support

Table 2.3—Characteristics of a Well-Functioning Health-Care Team

- Belief in the benefits of intensive diabetes management
- Respect for other team members, *including* the patient
- Appreciation for the value of patient–provider collaboration
- Participation in regular and ongoing communication among team members to provide consistent information to patients
- Ability to provide or to access multidisciplinary education and health-care expertise
- Availability of 24-hour assistance for problem solving

If the health-care team is not readily available or adequately prepared with the additional knowledge, skills, and resources necessary to implement intensive diabetes management or is not committed to utilization of this form of therapy, it would be better to refer patients wanting this approach to centers that are prepared to undertake this endeavor. Table 2.3 outlines the characteristics of well-functioning health-care team. A collaborative relationship between the diabetes team and the primary care provider is crucial to the success and effectiveness of the patient's treatment plan. This relationship is particularly important in view of the fact that the primary care provider is often the recipient of after-hours calls from patients.

DEFINING TEAM MEMBERS' ROLES

A clear understanding of the team's practice pattern and the responsibilities of individual team members is a key requirement for team functioning. Each member's contribution to the team effort should be determined by his or her educational background, credentials, individual abilities, experience, interests, and overall goals of team operation. Importantly, the multidisciplinary team has been described as providing complementary skills, more contact time for the assessment and treatment of patients, and assisting patients with learning diabetes self-care through consistent messages, repetition of information, reinforcement of self-care behaviors, and greater availability to deal with diabetes concerns that may arise. Typical roles and responsibilities for the physician, nurse, dietitian, and mental health professional members of the diabetes care team are listed in Table 2.4. Note that these roles have considerable overlap, and few roles are exclusive.

The team's effectiveness will be influenced by the ability of its members to collaborate through mutual respect, a shared philosophy of treatment, consistent goals for patient care, and regular communication. Within the multidisciplinary framework, no team member operates in isolation. Instead, expertise and strengths are combined to achieve comprehensive patient care. Multidisciplinary care serves to extend the scope and availability of assessment, intervention, follow-up, and treatment for the individual with diabetes.

Multidisciplinary diabetes management cannot be limited to those teams working within one department or one institution. Comprehensive team manage-

---

Table 2.4—Typical Roles and Responsibilities of the Diabetes Care Team Members

- Role of the prescriber
  - Establish medical diagnosis and define treatment
  - Provide rationale for treatment
  - Collaborate openly with the patient and team to design and implement a treatment plan
  - Oversee overall patient management
  - Provide patient/family support
- Role of the nurse educator and clinician
  - Provide self-care assessment
  - Oversee patient education: self-management skills, technical proficiency, and problem solving
  - Offer family education and assessment
  - Complement physician visits with more frequent contact: acute problem management and blood glucose pattern review
  - Provide patient and family support
- Role of the dietitian
  - Offer nutrition assessment
  - Provide specialized medical nutrition therapy and meal plan development
  - Complement physician visits with more frequent contact: meal plan integration or modification, compensatory adjustments for variable food intake and/or exercise, and blood glucose pattern review
  - Provide patient and family support
- Role of mental health professional
  - Elicit and address patient and family concerns and fears about treatment regimen and possible adverse events
  - Identify treatment obstacles
  - Identify sources of support in the patient's daily life
  - Provide patient/family support
  - Offer psychological assessment and treatment or referral as needed

---

ment also can operate in a team composed of members located at different sites. For this approach to be effective, emphasis must be placed on ongoing, accurate, and complete communication among the team members. Regardless of how the team is created, its members must share common treatment goals and cooperate in treatment decisions to minimize confusion and conflict for the patient (see the section Team Communication).

Providers practicing in situations with little access to multidisciplinary care will need to become knowledgeable in all aspects of intensive management, to the best of their ability.

TEAM COMMUNICATION

Effective team communication includes an understanding of how to engage with patients and the development of a consistent treatment message and approach (see Table 2.5). Conflicting messages from providers confuse patients and diminish treatment effectiveness.

Table 2.5—Fostering Effective Team Communication

- Have a common philosophy and message
- Create well-defined expectations
- Be flexible with regard to professional boundaries
- Share responsibility
- Show respect for each discipline
- Speak frequently to one another both prior to and following patient contact

Within treatment teams, role definitions and boundaries serve to define certain tasks. The complex nature of diabetes management necessitates flexibility in these boundaries, however, resulting in a blending of roles and sharing of responsibilities. Rigid boundaries that separate professional disciplines can result in a territorial approach to patient care and limit the possibility to meet the patient's needs if a particular team member is unavailable.

Team meetings provide an opportunity for members to readily communicate with each other and to maintain a focused approach to their health-care practices (see Table 2.6). If held on a regular basis, team meetings facilitate review of individual patient problems or progress, identify health-care system obstacles and patient care trends, and provide the forum for active problem solving. Team meetings also facilitate ongoing support among the health-care providers struggling with particularly difficult patient situations and decrease conflicts within the team. In the absence of regularly scheduled team meetings, an alternative communication strategy among team members must be identified (i.e., e-mail, voicemail, or conference calls) to ensure that the team works well together.

CONCLUSION

A multidisciplinary team approach to diabetes treatment is likely the best way to provide patients with a holistic approach to diabetes care—one that addresses the complex parts of day-to-day management. In the present health-care system, it is difficult for any single clinician to treat diabetes with its many comorbidities and challenging lifestyle recommendations. The team allows for more effective treat-

Table 2.6—Conducting Effective Team Meetings

- Maintain focus on common philosophy, goals, and mutual respect
- Review patient progress or problems
- Identify individual patient behaviors that can be targeted by the team to enhance treatment efficacy
- Identify health-care system or clinic trends
- Provide active, multidisciplinary problem solving
- Offer support for team members

ment by having a diverse staff that offers complementary skills and more contact time for assessment and treatment of patients, developing treatment relationships, and supporting patients in learning diabetes self-care. Furthermore, as the diabetes epidemic increases, primary care physicians more frequently manage complicated diabetes patients who present with many comorbidities. This increases the number of clinical concerns that need to be addressed during primary care visits and results in less available physician time to address each individual problem. Therefore, team members' increased availability to and familiarity with diabetes patients may be crucial to improving diabetes care.

BIBLIOGRAPHY

American Diabetes Association. Standards of medical care in diabetes–2016. *Diabetes Care* 2016;39(Suppl. 1):S1–S111

Anderson D, Christison-Lagay J. Diabetes self-management in a community health center: improving health behaviors and clinical outcomes for underserved patients. *Clin Diabetes* 2008;26:22–27

Brink SJ, Miller M, Moltz K. Education and multidisciplinary team care concepts for pediatric and adolescent diabetes mellitus. *J Pediatr Endocrinol Metab* 2002;15:1113–1130

Caravalho JY, Saylor CR. An evaluation of a nurse case-managed program for children with diabetes. *Pediatr Nurs* 2000;26:296–300, 328

Davidson MB. Effect of nurse-directed diabetes care in a minority population. *Diabetes Care* 2003;26:2281–2287

Diabetes Control and Complications Trial (DCCT) Study Group. The effect of intensive treatment of diabetes on the development and progression of long-term complications in insulin-dependent diabetes mellitus. *N Engl J Med* 1993;329:977–986

Funnell MM, Brown TL, Childs BP, Haas LB, Hosey GM, Jensen B, Maryniuk M, Peyrot M, Piette JD, Reader D, Siminerio LM, Weinger K, Weiss MA. National standards for diabetes self-management education. *Diabetes Care* 2008;31:S97–S104

Glasgow RE, Hiss RG, Anderson RM, Friedman NM, Hayward RA, Marrero DG, Taylor CB, Vinicor F. Report of the Health Care Delivery Work Group: behavioral research related to the establishment of a chronic disease model for diabetes care. *Diabetes Care* 2001;24:124–130

Hirsch IB. The status of the diabetes team. *Clin Diabetes* 1998;16:145–146

Lawson ML, Frank MR, Fry MK, Perlman K, Sochett EB, Daneman D. Intensive diabetes management in adolescents with type 1 diabetes: the importance of intensive follow-up. *J Pediatr Endocrinol Metab* 2000;13:79–84

Leicher SB, Dreelin E, Moore S. Integration of clinical psychology in the comprehensive diabetes care team. *Clin Diabetes* 2004;22:129–131

Lorenz RA, Bubb J, Davis D, Jacobson A, Jannasch K, Kramer J, Lipps J, Schlundt D. Changing behavior: practical lessons from the Diabetes Control and Complications Trial. *Diabetes Care* 1996;19:648–652

National Diabetes Education Program, National Institutes of Health. *Redesigning the Heath Care Team: Diabetes Prevention and Lifelong Management.* Bethesda, MD, U.S. Department of Health and Human Services, 2011

Renders CM, Valk GD, Griffin SJ, Wagner EH, van Eijk JT, Assendelft WJJ. Interventions to improve the management of diabetes in primary care, outpatient, and community settings: a systematic review. *Diabetes Care* 2001;24:1821–1833

Ritholz MD, Beverly EA, Abrahamson MJ, Brooks KM, Hultgren BA, Weinger K. Physicians' perceptions of the type 2 diabetes multi-disciplinary treatment team: a qualitative study. *Diabetes Educ* 2011;37:794–800

Rubin, R. Facilitating self-care in people with diabetes. *Diabetes Spect* 2001;14:55–57

UK Prospective Diabetes Study Group. Intensive blood glucose control with sulfonylureas or insulin compared with conventional treatment and risk of complications in patients with type 2 diabetes. *Lancet* 1998;352:837–853

University of California San Diego Diabetes Control and Complications Trial (DCCT) Team. Blended roles, shared responsibilities: DCCT nurses and dietitians. *Diabetes Spect* 1994;7:272–275

Wagner EH. The role of patient care teams in chronic disease management. *BMJ* 2000;320:569–572

Diabetes Self-Management Support and Education

Highlights

Integration of the Team Approach

Diabetes Continuing Education

Assessment

Instruction
   Environment
   Planning
   Content
   Sequencing of Diabetes Education
   Education Strategies

Motivation and Support

Action Planning

Evaluation

Documentation

Conclusion

Bibliography

DOI: 10.2337/9781580406321.03

Highlights
Diabetes Self-Management
Support and Education

■ The patient using intensive diabetes management must translate new information and skills into behavior change. Each interaction with the patient is an opportunity for the health-care provider to teach, reinforce, and encourage. The team approach is best exemplified when information is consistent among team members.

■ The patient's readiness to learn new information is a necessary component of any negotiated education plan. The individual will be most receptive when the education is relevant to his or her current needs. In addition, eliciting the patient's commitment to behavior change is another integral component of any education program.

■ Education assessment includes information about the patient's knowledge, skills, attitudes, and current diabetes care behaviors. The patient must possess a basic level of understanding before learning the more sophisticated aspects of intensive diabetes self-management.

■ Education is communication and requires careful planning and delivery of pertinent information. Education should be sequenced to build on existing knowledge. Teaching methods include the use of print and audiovisual media. These items must be content-appropriate, readable, and culturally sensitive.

■ Intensive diabetes management requires active patient involvement and problem solving. As part of their education, some individuals may need assistance in actively participating in their care.

■ Evaluating the success of patient education can be practical and quick. By using a series of "what-if" questions, the educator is able to assess the patient's problem-solving abilities.

■ Documenting and communicating key aspects of the education experience allows diabetes educators to share information with primary care and referring physicians and other health-care providers.

Diabetes Self-Management Support and Education

As the Diabetes Control and Complications Trial (DCCT) demonstrated, diabetes self-management support (DSMS) and diabetes self-management education and support (DSME/S) is integral to the success of an intensive management program. Patients embarking on the road to glycemic control must not only understand the complexities of diabetes and perform the necessary technical skills, but also have confidence in the management strategies and their self-management abilities. Intensive management requires patients to assume an active role in clinical decisions on a daily basis. To do this safely and effectively, patients need a supportive, knowledgeable, and accessible professional health-care team.

DSME/S is successful when patients are able to translate the information and skills into behavior change. Consequently, diabetes education is more than a lecture or two on how to control the disease. Instead, it is an ongoing program of assessment, instruction, support, negotiation, and evaluation delivered by a team of diabetes professionals.

INTEGRATION OF THE TEAM APPROACH

A coordinated team of professionals provides depth to the patient's DSME/S. The physician; nurse manager, educator, or clinician; dietitian; mental health professional; and the pharmacist and exercise physiologist all contribute particular skills and focus. The physician may create a team by referring to a community-based patient education program or to local diabetes educators. The American Diabetes Association (ADA) and the American Association of Diabetes Educators (AADE) maintain lists of nationally recognized or accredited education programs. Additionally, the American Association of Diabetes Educators (AADE) assists in locating local diabetes educators. The National Certification Board for Diabetes Educators keeps a roster of certified diabetes educators.

Diabetes education should never stand alone. Instead, it is a component of the care and management of the patient with diabetes. All members of the treatment team are teachers. Each contact with the patient is an opportunity to teach, reinforce, or evaluate the effect of teaching.

Information must be consistent across professionals. This consistency allows the patient to develop the necessary trust in the management plan and in the health-care providers. Education materials must be consistent in content. Consequently, each team member should know what the others are teaching.

DIABETES CONTINUING EDUCATION

Diabetes information should be taught with the understanding that learning about and adjusting to the condition is an ongoing process. One class or a series of classes at diagnosis does not confer lifelong "immunity." Instead, education should be viewed as a treatment that requires periodic boosters and lifelong learning.

Patients vary in their willingness or readiness to learn. At times, learner readiness is high, including when new research findings are released, when new medications are available, when complications occur, and when developmental changes arise. At these times, the educator should capitalize on these "teachable moments" because the patient's motivation and interest are peaking.

Ongoing DSMS also helps people with diabetes maintain effective self-management throughout a lifetime of diabetes as they face new challenges and as treatment advances become available. DSME/S helps patients optimize metabolic control, prevent and manage complications, and maximize quality of life in a cost-effective manner.

DSMS and DSME/S are the ongoing processes of facilitating the knowledge, skill, and ability necessary for self-care. This process incorporates the needs, goals, and life experiences of the person with diabetes. The overall objectives of DSMS and DSME/S are to support informed decision making, self-care behaviors, problem-solving, and active collaboration with the health-care team to improve clinical outcomes, health status, and quality of life in a cost-effective manner.

ASSESSMENT

The first step in developing an individual education plan is to gather information about the patient's current knowledge, skills, attitudes, behaviors, and environment. Because intensive management is so dependent on the patient's involvement and decision making, certain basic facts and skills are necessary. Table 3.1 lists the prerequisite information for patients entering an intensive management program. In addition to having this prerequisite information, the patient must accurately and safely perform certain self-management skills. These skills include

- using a blood glucose meter or continuous glucose monitoring (CGM) device;
- troubleshooting problems with glucose measurements;
- testing urine or blood ketones;
- record keeping or data management; and
- preparing and delivering insulin.

A careful education assessment includes the following:

- **Personal and socioeconomic information:** age; developmental stage; level of formal education; family composition; significant others; cultural, religious, and ethnic factors; resources; health insurance; and transportation

---

Table 3.1—Basic Facts for the Candidate for Intensive Diabetes Management

- Medication: insulin action or insulin regimens
- Rationale for self-monitoring of blood glucose: frequency of checking, goals, patterns
- A1C: monitoring frequency, goals
- Nutrition management
  - Healthy food choices
  - Role of major nutrients: effect on blood glucose levels
  - Carbohydrate counting
  - Sick-day management
  - Label reading
  - Dining out and convenience foods
- Effect of exercise
- Interaction of exercise, nutrition, and medication
- Hypoglycemia: causes, treatment, prevention
- Glucagon
- Identifying the dawn phenomenon
- Hyperglycemia: causes, treatment, prevention
- Ketoacidosis: causes, treatment, prevention
- Complications: causes, symptoms, prevention, monitoring
- Effect of daily living on diabetes control
  - Alcohol consumption
  - Work schedules
  - Traveling
  - Illness or medications and control

- **Diabetes information:** type and duration of diabetes, current and previous management approaches, acute and chronic complications, previous diabetes education, and successes as well as challenges with adherence
- **Other medical information:** height, weight, blood pressure, pertinent laboratory values (e.g., blood glucose, A1C, lipids, albumin), other illnesses, other medications, general health status, visual and hearing acuity, and motor skills
- **Lifestyle factors:** use of alcohol, tobacco, or other social drugs; physical activity; stressors; occupation; recreation; and social support systems
- **Nutrition information:** meal and snack times, locations, and typical foods; food preferences and intolerances; previous experience with "diets"; and previous nutrition education
- **Education factors:** learning style, literacy, native language, readiness to learn, decision-making skills, health information–seeking behaviors, technology preferences, health beliefs (e.g., locus of control, confidence, experience with other chronic illnesses, coping patterns, fears, concerns), ability and willingness to seek help, expectations of and capacity to deal with failure, assertiveness skills, organizational skills, response to an education plan, and motivators or barriers

Some questions to elicit the patient's beliefs and concerns are listed in Table 3.2.

Table 3.2—Eliciting the Patient's Beliefs

- What has been your experience with chronic health problems?
- How do you usually deal with success and failure?
- How has your diabetes affected your family?
- What worries or concerns you most about having diabetes?
- How do you typically learn new things?
- What one thing would you tell someone newly diagnosed with diabetes?
- What is the hardest part of diabetes management?
- What do you hope improved diabetes management will do for you?

INSTRUCTION

ENVIRONMENT

The learning environment includes not only the physical facility but also the characteristics of the instructor who facilitates the learning. To help the patient focus on the content, the location should be quiet, with adequate lighting, and free from distractions. Such attention to the environment decreases the cognitive load of efficient learning. Qualities of the teacher that promote learning are listed in Table 3.3.

The educator must draw from an extensive knowledge base while translating this knowledge into language understandable to the patient-learner. Furthermore, the educator must be able to adjust an educational agenda to meet the learner's needs. For example, the educator may have determined that the patient should hear about different insulin programs, whereas the patient may want to learn about counting carbohydrates. Adult learners always will focus on what the educa-

Table 3.3—Qualities and Competencies of the Teacher

- Possesses a knowledge base that is current and extensive
- Holds a personal belief that patients can learn
- Is empathetic
- Is nonjudgmental
- Is adaptable: flexible in using a variety of teaching approaches
- Has a sense of humor
- Is able to
  - individualize information
  - encourage questions
  - allow adequate time for patients to answer
  - use clear, simple, concrete explanations
  - sequence educational topics
  - involve others as needed
  - repeat and reinforce facts
  - provide for reflection and review of content
  - evaluate understanding
  - provide focused and timely feedback

tion encounter will mean to them. The educator is most successful when able to adapt to changes in the teaching agenda.

Education is a process of communication and reception of information. Throughout the education session, the educator assesses the learner's understanding. By asking the patient to restate the information or to use the information to solve a problem, the educator is then able to evaluate learning.

PLANNING

As the assessment proceeds, the educator will identify topics and teaching approaches that are most appropriate for the patient. Shared goal setting is important. The plan for the education program becomes a negotiation between the teacher and learner.

Often, the patient doesn't know what he or she needs to know and may be resistant to new information. The educator's job is to gently challenge the patient's knowledge while presenting new information. The educator may need to remind the patient that medical knowledge about diabetes changes rapidly and old information is being replaced with new ways of handling the disease.

The educator's job is to engage the patient-learner in the education by building trust and listening to the learner's needs. The patient is more likely to remain interested when the content is meaningful and consistent with what the patient already knows. Strategies to maintain interest include using interactive teaching approaches and incorporating time for review and reflection of new content.

CONTENT

Topics especially pertinent for the patient implementing intensive diabetes management include

- nutrition guidelines and the effect of food on glycemic control,
- insulin action and dosage adjustment,
- impact of exercise on blood glucose control,
- monitoring,
- prevention and detection of chronic complications,
- behavior change strategies, and
- problem solving.

A comprehensive curriculum list is included in Table 3.4.

SEQUENCING OF DIABETES EDUCATION

There is far too much information on intensive management to deliver in one session. Effective diabetes education occurs over several contacts with the patient. The most meaningful education sessions build on the patient's existing knowledge and on content from previous sessions. For instance, one session may be devoted to a discussion about insulin regimens, the interpretation of blood glucose results, and recordkeeping. The next session may focus on problem solving by reviewing blood glucose records and discussing and demonstrating insulin adjustment techniques.

Table 3.4—Curriculum for Intensive Management

- Diabetes overview and review
  - DCCT results: long-term control and benefits
  - Benefits, risks, and management options for improving glucose control
- Stress and psychosocial adjustment
  - Effect of stress on control
  - Identifying stressors
  - Anticipating stress
  - Problem solving: stress management techniques
- Family involvement and social support
  - Sharing diabetes care: when and how
  - Seeking help
  - Joining support groups
  - Doing volunteer work
- Nutrition
  - Role of nutrients
  - Glycemic impact
  - Label reading
  - Advanced carbohydrate counting or other meal-planning approach
  - Alcohol: effect and use
  - Dining out versus cooking in (adapting recipes)
  - Problem solving: evaluating the effect of food adjustments and changes
- Exercise and activity
  - Effect of exercise
  - Exercise physiology
  - Prolonged effect, late postexercise hypoglycemia
  - Planning pre-exercise food or insulin
  - Problem solving: evaluating effect of exercise
- Diabetes medication
  - Insulin: preparation, injection, storage, site selection
  - Insulin delivery systems: technical training for use of pens and pumps
  - Problem solving: insulin dose changes
    - Using results of monitoring to evaluate blood glucose patterns and variability
    - Basal changes
    - Bolus changes (i.e., algorithms)
    - Supplemental doses or sensitivity factors
    - Evaluating and verifying the effect of dose adjustment
    - When to call the diabetes team
- Monitoring
  - Blood glucose meter use: technique, meter care, troubleshooting
  - Fingerstick or alternative site technique, care of skin
  - Continuous glucose monitoring
  - Recordkeeping and data management
  - Understanding and using glucose results
  - When to check urine or blood ketones, and interpretation of results
  - Relationship among nutrition, exercise, medication, and blood glucose levels
  - Effect of unusual days on glucose control
    - Travel
    - Varying work schedules
  - Anticipating changes and making adjustments
- Prevention, detection, and treatment of acute complications
  - Identifying symptoms and causes of hypoglycemia
  - Understanding how symptoms may change as glycemic control improves

Table 3.4— Curriculum for Intensive Management (*Continued*)

- • Glucagon: when to use, who to train, precautions
- • Symptoms and causes of hyperglycemia and its management
- • Diabetic ketoacidosis
■ Prevention, detection, and treatment of chronic complications
  - • Detection of problems: routine health follow-up and diabetes-specific follow-up
  - • Effect of intensification on existing complications
  - • Foot, skin, and dental care
    - - Injection sites
    - - Prevention of infections
    - - Dental prophylaxis
■ Behavior change strategies, goal setting, negotiation skills, and problem solving
  - • Decision-making skills
  - • Problem-solving approaches
  - • Interacting with diabetes team
■ Preconception, pregnancy, and postpartum management
■ Use of health-care systems and community resources
  - • Creating a diabetes management team
  - • Financial impact and cost-saving strategies for intensive diabetes management

EDUCATION STRATEGIES

Adults learn best when the information is immediately useful and relevant. Thus, teaching a patient to implement an intensive management plan must include enough time to practice the decision making required and focus on information needed to implement the treatment plan. For example, if the patient will be using an algorithm to adjust insulin doses, then the educator must plan for opportunities to practice using that algorithm.

The educator should have a repertoire of real-life examples to use when teaching. Most individuals need help to develop the judgment and problem solving needed to make diabetes decisions. Consider, for instance, what a patient must evaluate in choosing an insulin dose before a meal. How much carbohydrate and fat will be consumed? What is the current blood glucose level? How far from target is the blood glucose level? What range of insulin doses tends to work for this mealtime? What will the exercise level be in the next couple of hours? How long should the time between injection and meal be? Working through several examples with the patient allows the educator to model good decision making. Decision-making and problem-solving skills are acquired and improved through practice. Mistakes are part of the learning process. The educator must create opportunities for practice and an environment in which errors and misjudgments are used to learn, not criticize.

Other approaches include using print, audiovisual, and web-based materials. Many excellent materials are available from manufacturers of diabetes supplies. These materials, however, must be evaluated individually for appropriate content, readability, and cultural sensitivity. Interactive educational materials—for example, computer programs, food models, self-instructional materials, and games—

Table 3.5—Sample Worksheet for Intensive Diabetes Management

Goals for Intensive Blood Glucose Control

	ADA guidelines	*Personal goals*
Preprandial plasma glucose	80–130 mg/dL (4.4–7.2 mmol/L)	_____ to _____
Peak postprandial glucose	<180 mg/dL (<10.0 mmol/L) 2 h after the start of a meal	Below _____
A1C	<7%	

Basal Insulin

Time	*Type*	*Dose*

Bolus Insulin

Time	*Type*	*Dose*	*Carbohydrate Amount*

Carbhydrate-to-Insulin Ratio: Breakfast: _____; Lunch: _____; Dinner: _____; Bedtime: _____

Correction Insulin Dose: _____ units for every _____ mg/dL blood glucose

add variety to the education program and enhance learner engagement in the process. A sample patient education handout is provided in Table 3.5.

Regardless of the methodology for instruction, one of the most effective approaches to encouraging adherence is simple: Provide the literate patient with clear, written instructions. Patients generally remember very little from their time with the clinician or educator. Written instructions can be the educator's most practical tool.

MOTIVATION AND SUPPORT

The process of patient education is intimately connected to behavior change. The educator should assess how the patient will use or transfer the information to action. Simply asking the patient, "How will you try this at home?" or "What things will be easy or hard to do?" often will alert the educator to potential diffi-

Table 3.6—Verifying the Patient's Commitment

- How effective do you think this task will be for you?
- What part of the plan may be hard for you?
- Are you concerned about the time or expense?
- How will you know if the plan is working?
- How certain are you that you can do this?
- What makes you certain or uncertain?
- If now is not the right time for you to begin, when will the time be right?

culties in adherence. Some questions to elicit the patient's commitment to behavior change are listed in Table 3.6.

ACTION PLANNING

Some patients have adequate diabetes knowledge and wish to participate in their care, but they lack the assertive communication or negotiation skills needed. They may feel intimidated by the health-care professional or by the system. Yet, patient involvement in treatment decisions is important for the individual on an intensive management program. Because the patient will direct so much of the daily management, his or her commitment to the plan is essential.

The educator may assess commitment and confidence with a simple rating tool. After developing an action plan with the patient, the educator asks the patient to rate how confident he or she feels in following the plan. The patient then rates confidence on a scale of 1 to 10 (1 being not at all confident; 10 being highly confident). The educator then should explore what supports the chosen rating and what is preventing a higher rating. Such exploration reveals motivators or supports as well as barriers to behavior change.

The educator may find that the patient actually needs assistance in communicating his or her needs to the physician. The patient's education plan may include tips on how to participate actively in the treatment plan.

EVALUATION

Often in a busy practice, patient education amounts to nothing more than the professional relaying information, with little time directed at assessing how the information is received and implemented. Whether provided in the physician's office or in a formal classroom education setting, evaluating the success of patient education can be quick and easy.

Tests and quizzes have a place in some education programs. The adult learner, however, will remember information that is immediately useful. Education sessions should include sufficient time for reflection on the material discussed. Questions to promote reflection and review are listed in Table 3.7. Using a series of "what-if" questions allows the educator not only to assess level of knowledge but

Table 3.7—Providing Reflection and Review of Educational Content

- What are the three most important points?
- What questions do you still have?
- What did you find most interesting?
- What did you find most difficult?
- How would you summarize this content?
- How could you learn more about this topic?
- What did you learn that was new to you?
- What do you want always to remember?
- How does this content relate to something you already know?
- What will help you remember this material?
- What did you find most surprising?
- What will be the hardest thing to remember?
- How will you use what you learned today?
- What content will make the most difference for you?

also to determine problem-solving abilities. A sample of such questions is provided in Table 3.8.

DOCUMENTATION

The diabetes educator is obligated to completely document the education process from assessment through evaluation. Checklists and documentation forms may be created to assist the educator in this task. Sample forms are provided in the section on Education Recognition Program at http://professional.diabetes.org. To provide continuity and consistency and to facilitate the team approach, the educator, in addition to documenting the medical record, also should provide follow-up information to the referring physician or prescriber.

Table 3.8—Evaluating Learning and Problem Solving

- What would you do if
  - you gave yourself insulin and your restaurant meal was late?
  - you were supposed to take rapid-acting insulin before a meal, but your blood glucose level was 40 mg/dL?
  - you were planning to exercise 1 h after lunch?
  - you awakened with nausea and did not feel like eating?
  - your blood glucose results did not coincide with how you felt?
- How will you adjust your management plan for special occasions and parties?

CONCLUSION

Patient education is integral to the success of intensifying the individual's diabetes management. The patient must be skilled, knowledgeable, and willing to participate fully and successfully in the decisions about daily self-care. The physician, diabetes educators, and other professionals must form a unified patient care team to ensure that the patient receives consistent and accurate information. Providing DSMS and DSMS/E requires attention to patient assessment, individual instruction, and evaluation of patient response and the patient's willingness to participate in their care.

BIBLIOGRAPHY

American Association of Diabetes Educators (AADE). *The Art and Science of Diabetes Self-Management Education: A Desk Reference for Healthcare Professionals.* 3rd ed. Chicago, AADE, 2014

American Diabetes Association. *Medical Management of Type 1 Diabetes.* 6th ed. Kaufman F, Ed. Alexandria, VA, American Diabetes Association, 2012

Anderson B, Funnel M. *The Art of Empowerment: Stories and Strategies for Diabetes Educators.* 2nd ed. Alexandria, VA, American Diabetes Association, 2005

Bodenheimer T, Davis C, Holman H. Helping patients adopt healthier behaviors. *Clin Diabetes* 2007;25:66–70

Boren SA, Fitzner AK, Panhalkar PS, Specker J. Costs and benefits associated with diabetes education: a review of the literature. *Diabetes Educ* 2009;31(1):72–96

Burke SD, Sherr D, Lipman RD. Partnering with diabetes educators to improve patient outcomes. *Diabetes Metab Syndr Obes* 2014;2:45–53

Childs B, Cypress M, Spollett G (Eds.). *Complete Nurse's Guide to Diabetes Care.* 2nd ed. Alexandria, VA, American Diabetes Association, 2009

Dick W, Carey L, Carey JO. *The Systematic Design of Instruction.* 8th ed. Boston, Pearson, 2015

Duncan I, Ahmed T, Li Q, Stetson B, Ruggiero L, Burton K, Rosenthal D, Fitzner K. Assessing the value of the diabetes educator. *Diabetes Educ* 2011;37:638–657

Gardner, H. *Multiple Intelligences: New Horizons.* New York, Perseus Books Group, 2006

Gary TL, Genkinger JM, Guallar E, Peyrot M, Brancati FL. Meta-analysis of randomized educational and behavioral interventions in type 2 diabetes. *Diabetes Educ* 2003;29:488–501

Haas LL, Maryniuk M, Beck J, Cox CE, Duker P, Edwards L, Fisher EB, Hanson
    L, Kent D, Kolb L, McLaughlin S, Orzeck E, Piette JD, Rhinehart AS, Roth-
    man R, Sklaroff S, Tomky D, Youseff G. National standards for diabetes self-
    management education and support. *Diabetes Care* 2014;37(Suppl. 1):
    S144–S153

King EB, Schlundt DG, Pichert JW, Kinzer CK, Backer BA. Improving the skills
    of health professionals in engaging patients in diabetes-related problem solv-
    ing. *J Contin Educ Health Prof* 2002;22:94–102

Mensing C. Comparing the processes: Accreditation and recognition. *Diabetes
    Spect* 2010;23:65–78

Norris SL, Lau J, Smith SJ, Schmid CH, Engelgau MM. Self-management educa-
    tion for adults with type 2 diabetes: a meta-analysis of the effect on glycemic
    control. *Diabetes Care* 2002;25:1159–1171

Rollnick S, Miller WR, Butler CC. *Motivational Interviewing in Health Care*. New
    York, Guilford Press, 2008

Psychosocial Issues

DOI: 10.2337/9781580406321.04

Highlights
Psychosocial Issues

- Active patient engagement with self-care behaviors and the willingness to collaborate on treatment decisions are good indicators of future success with an intensive diabetes management plan. Patient engagement is promoted by an effective patient–clinician relationship and communication. From the outset of treatment, clinicians need to foster patients' active inquiry and participation so that self-care behaviors can be discussed, monitored for mastery and effectiveness, and modified in an ongoing fashion.

- Understanding and addressing the psychosocial factors that may promote or interfere with patients' active engagement in intensive diabetes management is of critical importance. Therefore, psychosocial assessments are needed both before intensification of diabetes management begins and throughout the course of treatment. Diabetes burnout, diabetes distress, depression, anxiety, eating disorders, and substance abuse may interfere with patients' intensive diabetes management and need to be assessed and monitored when patients display difficulties with their intensive management. Thus, the clinician can have increased understanding of the possible reasons for the patients' behavior and, with the assistance of the multidisciplinary treatment team, can begin an effective treatment.

- Clinicians should be aware that depression, diabetes distress, and eating disorders are prevalent in patients with diabetes. As a way to address these psychosocial concerns, clinicians should consider using diabetes-specific screening surveys for diabetes distress or non-diabetes-specific surveys for depression. If screening identifies existing problems, further evaluation by a qualified mental health professional is indicated. The mental health professional may use cognitive-behavioral, interpersonal, or family counseling approaches to assist patients with psychosocial difficulties. In addition, the mental health professional must be included as a member of the multidisciplinary treatment team, which is critically important when engaging the patient with psychosocial difficulties in intensive diabetes treatment.

■ Periods of psychological distress are expected in the life course of diabetes. For example, how patients perceive and manage the specter or onset of diabetes complications is important to assess. Patients' negative emotional responses and attitudes toward complications may result in their loss of desire for intensive management. These responses may interact with treatment goals and affect intensive management. Importantly, clinicians need to recognize that these reactions are expected and normative, and patients need support in adapting to their actual or perceived limitations. Furthermore, negative responses should be monitored and addressed, especially if they are continuing for too long a period of time.

■ Patients are more likely to succeed with self-care regimens that are responsive to their lifestyle needs and do not present an overwhelming burden. Therefore, patients should be encouraged to set treatment goals that can best fit their personal lifestyle. These goals should be collaboratively determined by patient and clinician and thereby should be achievable by the patient. Ensure that patients begin intensive treatment by feeling they can meet their goals rather than by setting goals that are too difficult to accomplish, which may lead to self-blame, discouragement, and a sense of failure. Furthermore, periodic lapses in self-care behaviors should be accepted as an expected part of intensive diabetes management. Patients may become tired of the demands of intensive diabetes management, resulting in burnout. Therefore, ongoing monitoring and support from health-care professionals are essential to the achievement and maintenance of treatment goals.

Psychosocial Issues

U se of intensive diabetes management during the Diabetes Control and Complications Trial (DCCT) demonstrated that patients can and will follow a medical regimen that is complex and multifaceted when provided with extensive education and professional support. In the more than 20 years since the DCCT results, intensive diabetes management has become the gold standard treatment for most patients with type 1 diabetes (T1D) and for many with type 2 diabetes (T2D) who use insulin. The Look AHEAD study also showed that when multidisciplinary services are available, user friendly, and personalized, a high degree of adherence with a complex lifestyle-based regimen could be achieved and sustained, and intensive treatment goals for T2D could be met without detrimental effects to the patient's quality of life.

Consequently, health-care professionals need to spend time presenting a background of the benefits and barriers for intensive treatment. By discussing the DCCT and more recent studies, clinicians can promote patients' increased understanding of the importance of active involvement with self-care behaviors and collaboration in treatment decisions, which are good indicators of future success with an intensive management plan.

Most important, patients' active engagement is necessary for successful diabetes management. To promote this engagement, glucose targets and treatment goals should include and reflect the patient's needs, preferences, and values. Furthermore, understanding and addressing the psychosocial factors that may promote or interfere with patients' active engagement in intensive diabetes management is of critical importance. Thus, psychosocial assessments are needed both before intensive diabetes management begins and throughout the course of treatment. Moreover, active patient engagement requires an effective patient–clinician relationship and open communication to support intensive diabetes management.

PSYCHOSOCIAL ASSESSMENT

PSYCHOLOGICAL FACTORS

Psychological distress or well-being can affect a patient's ability to carry out the behavior and communication necessary to implement and maintain intensive diabetes management. Evaluation of current and prior psychological status by a mental health professional familiar with diabetes should be included with the assessment of the patient's physical status. These evaluations should be an integral and ongoing part of intensive diabetes management. The easiest and most direct methods involve short, standardized screening surveys that can identify psychological factors that might interfere with patients' optimal engagement in intensive diabetes management. Some examples of surveys for diabetes distress include Problem Areas in Diabetes (PAID) and the Diabetes Distress Scale (DDS). Some widely used although not diabetes-specific surveys for depression include the Patient Health Questionnaire 9 (PHQ-9) and the Center for Epidemiological Studies Depression Scale (CES-D). If screening identifies problems, further evaluation by a qualified mental health professional is indicated. When referral to a mental health professional is made, always include this professional in the treatment team. This professional can help with treatment decisions and assist family members and others (such as teachers, friends, or coworkers) to support needed behaviors and attitude changes.

A potential contraindication to intensification is the prior or current diagnosis of a psychiatric illness that impairs an individual's ability to carry out activities of daily living (including diabetes self-care tasks). In addition, clinicians also should consider assessing whether the patient can

- make, evaluate, or implement treatment decisions;
- use appropriate problem-solving skills; and
- maintain close contact with a clinician.

If the patient is found to have deficits in the any of these areas, then appropriate psychosocial supports, such as a mental health professional to provide counseling or a case manager to monitor adverse treatment outcomes (e.g., repeated diabetic ketoacidosis [DKA]) should be put in place before intensified treatment begins.

Diabetes Burnout

Intensive management places greater burdens on the patient than conventional treatment approaches and therefore may contribute to the potential for diabetes burnout, diabetes distress, depression, and reduced quality of life. The occurrence of complications that produce functional limitations, such as worsening eyesight or decreased mobility resulting from micro- and macrovascular disease, also can be sources of diabetes burnout. Therefore, it is important that clinicians assess patients for burnout through the course of treatment. Some important ways to address diabetes burnout include referral to a mental health professional, meeting with other diabetes patients in support groups, and bringing in the patient's family to help them understand what the patient is feeling and how they can support him or her.

Diabetes Distress and Depression

Studies have shown that many patients with diabetes who display high levels of depressive symptoms also experience high levels of emotional distress stemming from concerns and worries associated with their diabetes and its management. As a result, diabetes distress should be considered to understand and treat the emotional distresses that patients with diabetes manifest. Emotional distress is a single, continuous dimension that includes both content (diabetes and its management and other life stresses) and severity, both of which can be addressed directly in clinical care.

The relationship between depression and diabetes appears to be bidirectional, that is, each may contribute to the other. Depression in individuals with diabetes has been implicated in nonadherence with self-care behaviors, lack of motivation to intensify treatment, reduced quality of life, and worsened glycemia. It is believed that depression is underdiagnosed in the diabetes population, and importantly, the American Diabetes Association (ADA) recommends that older adults (>65 years of age) with diabetes should be considered a high-priority population for depression screening and treatment. When assessing patients, health-care professionals need to be alert to the following situations, which may contribute to patients' distress or depression:

- Diagnosis of diabetes
- Adverse effects of treatment (e.g., severe hypoglycemia, weight gain, or perceived treatment failure)
- Onset of complications
- Negative effect of diabetes care on lifestyle
- Lack of real or perceived support in the home, work, school, or other social environment
- Change in real or perceived self-image or functional abilities
- Fluctuations in physical well-being and mood associated with changes in glucose levels
- Increased burden, including finances, of medical care

Anxiety

Increased anxiety in people with diabetes can occur at diabetes diagnosis, key life transitions (going to college, getting married, starting first job, pregnancy), and the onset of complications. Fear of hypoglycemia is the most common severe anxiety for people with diabetes, which can lead patients to maintain blood glucose levels above recommended targets, increasing their risk for diabetes complications. Many people with diabetes and depression also have comorbid anxiety disorders, such as generalized anxiety disorder, panic disorder, or posttraumatic stress disorder. Anxiety disorders also can occur without comorbid depression in people with diabetes. Anxiety disorders may complicate diabetes management in the following ways: *1*) distinguishing between feelings of anxiety and symptoms of hypoglycemia may make it difficult to know how and when to respond appropriately to distressing feelings; *2*) preexisting anxiety may lead to severe anxiety or panic disorders after a person is diagnosed with diabetes and needs to begin using injections or have blood draws; and *3*) fear of hypoglycemia can lead some patients to maintain blood glucose levels above the target range.

Fear of hypoglycemia. More frequent episodes of hypoglycemia can be expected when blood glucose levels hover around the normal range, the goal of intensive management. Individuals vary significantly regarding their risk for hypoglycemia, their ability to recognize hypoglycemia symptoms, and their adaptive behaviors for coping with hypoglycemia as well as the social support they receive for monitoring, recognizing, and treating episodes of hypoglycemia. Furthermore, the overlap between symptoms of hypoglycemia and anxiety can make recognition of episodes difficult. Some patients may develop a maladaptive fear of hypoglycemia that leads them to actively avoid target glucose levels, which is counterproductive to intensive management. Although training patients, families, and others to recognize and treat hypoglycemia or severe hypoglycemia in their home or work environment is usually part of basic diabetes education, this issue should be revisited whenever diabetes management is intensified.

Patients learn to fear hypoglycemia not only for the potential adverse physical outcomes, but also for the lack of control that results from neuroglycopenia (low glucose in the brain). Patients experiencing hypoglycemia may act silly, risqué, angry, or irresponsible; take risks or withdraw. Altered personality characteristics are common. Low blood glucose levels can affect interactions with partners and coworkers, cause errors in mental processing, or alter physical functioning (e.g., cause automobile accidents), all of which are beyond the control of the patient during a hypoglycemic episode.

Fear of hypoglycemia should be periodically assessed, especially if patients' HbA_{1c} is above target levels. When questioned, a patient may describe inappropriately eliminating or excessively reducing insulin doses in relation to the perceived risk of hypoglycemia. In this situation, patients may 1) fear an abrupt drop in blood glucose level even if their blood glucose is well above 70 mg/dL, 2) misinterpret feelings of anxiety as hypoglycemia and inappropriately treat the hypoglycemia without addressing the anxiety, 3) develop heightened fear following an episode of severe hypoglycemia or after repeated episodes of hypoglycemia, and 4) aim for a relatively high blood glucose range, above which they feel safer from the risk of hypoglycemia.

Some suggested options for addressing fear of hypoglycemia include the following: 1) use of continuous subcutaneous insulin pump therapy or continuous glucose monitoring (CGM); 2) teach strategies to increase recognition of symptoms; 3) prevent low blood glucose by temporarily reducing insulin doses; and 4) increase the frequency of blood glucose monitoring (e.g., before and after exercise, before driving). Studies indicate that CGM can positively influence hypoglycemia management by decreasing spouses' anxiety, vigilance, and negative experiences. If fear of hypoglycemia becomes an impediment to achieving optimal glycemia, refer the patient to a mental health professional who specializes in diabetes. Behavioral techniques such as exposure in cases in which patients learn to tolerate lower blood glucose levels in the presence of a therapist or family member are effective strategies.

Needle phobia. Many individuals who must use insulin initially express fear of taking injections but quickly accommodate, out of necessity, to giving themselves insulin. In most cases, firm expectations for the patient's behavior (along with social support and skill building) effectively reduce fear and anxiety. When anxiety and avoidant behaviors increase around giving injections, needle phobia may be the underlying cause. Avoidant behaviors can include, but are not limited to, rituals that prolong the period before the injection is given, intense expressions of distress (moaning, crying, yelling) accompanied by physical withdrawal from the needle, or frank refusal to take injections.

When needle phobia is suspected, an evaluation by a qualified mental health professional is indicated. Cognitive-behavioral therapy, relaxation techniques, and pharmacotherapy are effective in reducing phobic behavior. Insulin pump therapy also can be considered, although pump malfunctions will still require the use of occasional injections and the actual infusion set may be feared. Regardless of the intervention strategies used, it is important that the patient receive pragmatic and nonjudgmental messages about the necessity of overcoming these fears. At the same time, health-care professionals need to acknowledge the degree of distress the patient is experiencing so that appropriate psychological treatment can occur.

Importantly, include significant others in the behavioral intervention because the patient's anxious behaviors may be inadvertently supported, encouraged, and maintained within the context of family dynamics. A prime example of this is a parent who grimaces and cries every time the child with diabetes receives an injection. The child learns to associate negative emotions and distress with receiving an injection even though he or she may experience little physical pain. In these circumstances, needle phobia may evolve. Thus, the child attempts to avoid a "feared stimulus" and also receives parental support for the avoidant behavior. Therefore, both parent and child would benefit from the behavioral intervention.

Psychological insulin resistance. Psychological insulin resistance is sometimes seen when patients with T2D must begin using insulin. This reaction to beginning insulin may include needle phobia, unreasonable personal beliefs about the meaning of insulin therapy, poor self-efficacy, and a lack of accurate information. Patients also may perceive that starting insulin means that she or he has "failed" diabetes management. Importantly, clinicians need to stop using the start of insulin as a threat to motivate patients' improved self-care, because this message implies blame or failure in self-management behavior if and when insulin becomes part of treatment. Suggestions for addressing the start of insulin include helping the patient understand the progressive course of diabetes, demonstrating how oral medication may not be working anymore, and discussing insulin injections as a powerful and necessary tool to achieve glycemic targets.

Eating Disorders

Type 1 diabetes and eating disorders. Studies suggest an increased risk of eating disorders among female patients with T1D. Intermittent insulin restriction for weight-loss purposes has been found to be a common practice among women with T1D. For example, in women and girls with T1D between the ages of 13 and 60 years, 31% reported intentional insulin restriction. Rates of restriction peaked in late adolescence and early adulthood, with 40% of women and girls between the ages of 15 and 30 years reporting intentional restriction. Furthermore, eating problems are reported to continue to increase past age 30 years.

Even at a subclinical level of severity, restricting insulin places women at heightened risk for the medical complications of diabetes. Women reporting intentional insulin restriction had higher A1C levels (by as much as 2 or more points), more frequent hospital and emergency room visits, greater episodes of DKA, and higher rates of neuropathy and retinopathy than women who did not report insulin restriction. Insulin restriction was found to triple the risk of mortality during an 11-year follow-up study. Most important, women who stopped insulin restriction reported thinking differently about insulin and weight; no longer fearing that healthy glycemia and appropriate insulin treatment would automatically lead to weight gain.

Although the large majority of research on eating disorders and T1D focuses on insulin restriction as a central symptom, not all patients with eating disorders and T1D restrict insulin. For example, patients with anorexia and T1D require significantly less insulin than usual by virtue of severe calorie restriction and related weight loss. Their eating disorder may go undetected for a while because their glucose values are likely to be in or below the target range. It may not be until they reach a notably low weight or develop a pattern of recurrent hypoglycemia, that their eating disorder is discovered. Additionally, patients with bulimia and T1D may not always use insulin restriction to purge calories. For example, they may self-induce vomiting or turn to excessive exercise and other means of purging. These behaviors may not have as strong an impact on glycemia as insulin restriction—possibly making eating disorder detection more difficult in these patients as well.

Clinicians may find it helpful to use screening tools to identify patients with eating disorders or those at risk. The Diabetes Eating Problem Survey–Revised (DEPS-R) is a 16-item self-report questionnaire that takes <10 min to complete. The five-item mSCOFF survey has been adapted to help identify insulin restriction and eating disorder behavior.

Type 2 diabetes and binge eating. Because obesity is a significant risk factor in T2D, recurrent binge eating may increase the chances of developing this form of diabetes. Research indicates that a distinct subgroup of obese adults (20–46%) engage in recurrent binge eating.

The literature on binge eating in T2D has grown in recent years. 14% of the patients with newly diagnosed T2D experienced problems with binge eating, compared with 4% of the age-, sex-, and weight-matched control subjects. Participants in the Look AHEAD study who stopped binge eating were found to be able to lose similar amounts of weight when compared with those who did not report binge eating. Participants with binge eating disorder were younger than participants without eating disorders and reported that their weight problems began at younger ages. These data raise the possibility that recurrent binge eating is a risk factor for developing T2D earlier in life. In fact, in the TODAY Study, which evaluated treatments for T2D in adolescence, participants who endorsed problems with binge eating had higher rates of extreme obesity.

Treatment recommendations. The International Conference on Eating Disorders and Diabetes Mellitus Guidelines recommend a multidisciplinary team approach, including an endocrinologist or diabetologist, nurse educator, nutritionist with eating disorder or diabetes training, and psychologist or social worker with eating disorder expertise to provide weekly individual therapy. Depending on the level of comorbid depression and anxiety, a psychiatrist may be needed for psychopharmacological evaluation and treatment. Treatment outcome research in eating disorders in the general population supports using cognitive-behavioral therapy in combination with antidepressant medications as the most effective treatment. These approaches need to be adapted to directly address the role of insulin restriction for those patients with this symptom.

Once established as a longstanding behavior pattern, the problem of frequent insulin restriction may be particularly difficult to treat. For this reason, early detection and intervention appears to be crucial. Disordered eating behaviors often are associated with intense shame and secrecy and thus identifying disordered eating as a common struggle in T1D can help the patient with feelings of isolation and to decrease shame. As for all patients, build a close patient–clinician relationship characterized by open communication and a nonjudgmental stance. This may make it more likely for the patient to feel comfortable disclosing the problem and turning to the diabetes treatment team for help.

With active insulin restriction, the treatment team must be willing to set incremental goals that the patient feels ready to achieve. The first goal is to establish medical safety by focusing on the prevention of DKA and the acute onset of complications. Early in treatment, intensive glycemic management of diabetes is not an appropriate target. The DCCT and other studies have shown that rapid A1C improvement in individuals with longstanding hyperglycemia can be associated with rapid progression of retinopathy and severe, treatment-induced neuropathy. Therefore, ophthalmologists and neurologists recommend slowly improving glycemia in these patients; however, there are no clinical guidelines regarding optimal rates for improving glycemic control. Gradually, the team can build toward increased doses of insulin, increases in food intake, greater flexibility in meal plans, regularity of eating routines, more frequent blood glucose monitoring, and the final goal of intensive diabetes management.

Substance Abuse

Alcohol consumption is inversely associated with glycemic targets among diabetes patients and is a marker for poorer adherence to diabetes self-care behaviors. In a study of adolescents with chronic illnesses including T1D, it was found that alcohol and marijuana use are prevalent among youth with chronic medical conditions and that alcohol use was associated with youth who reported regularly forgetting to take their medications. Thus, both before beginning intensive diabetes management and during the course of treatment, it is important for health-care providers to inquire and educate adolescent and adult patients about alcohol use and the ways that it may interfere with and impede diabetes self-care and optimal glycemia.

Stress

Stressors—positive and negative, long or short term—affect the individual's ability to maintain optimal glycemia. The patient's response to stress should be assessed before intensive treatment is begun to identify regimen strategies that will best maximize individual methods of coping with stress. The identification of stress-related events and symptoms is important in identifying potential causes of high or fluctuating blood glucose levels. One possible impact of stress on diabetes management relates to its way of disrupting daily routines and sometimes realigning priorities for a time. These changes not only influence glucose, but also the physiological impact of stress has an additional potential effect on glycemia. Furthermore, transient stress causes a state of relative insulin resistance as a result of increased concentrations of counterregulatory hormones and leads to hyperglycemia. The effects of chronic stress on glycemia are not well understood.

Health-care professionals can help patients evaluate the effects of stressful life events through the use of careful blood glucose–monitoring records in which the patient is encouraged to record life events as well as blood glucose level and insulin dose. The patient can learn how to distinguish symptoms caused by life stress, which in turn may affect blood glucose levels, from symptoms that might be expected from more normative changes in blood glucose levels (e.g., feelings of hunger and light-headedness before a planned meal). Patients practicing intensive management should be encouraged to check blood glucose whenever they feel symptoms or experience psychosocial stress to identify their own pattern of glycemic response. With use of CGM, this is easier to do because of frequency of glucose readings and the ability to identify patterns.

Although stressful lifestyles do not preclude an intensive diabetes management regimen, a patient must learn to cope effectively with changes in blood glucose levels caused by stress and to develop and practice coping behaviors. Intervention strategies for stress reduction can include relaxation techniques, regular exercise regimens, support people or groups, medications, and changes in the diabetes management regimen. Intervention strategies should be tailored to the source of the stress, the patient's glycemic response, and the resources (psychological and other) the patient possesses to cope with the stressor.

Patterns of eating in response to stress also need to be addressed for individuals with both T1D and T2D. Patients need counseling to develop coping skills for maintaining glucose levels within the acceptable range through exercise, insulin, or medication modifications when stress-related or emotional eating is identified. Identification of stressors that impede maintenance of optimal glycemia and the development of coping strategies may best be achieved with the help of a mental health professional familiar with diabetes who is integrated into the diabetes care team.

Diabetes Complications

When meeting with patients who have diabetes, discuss the results of the DCCT and its follow-up study, Epidemiology of Diabetes Interventions and Complications (EDIC), which found that intensive treatment targeting near-normal glycemia delays the onset and slows the progression of serious diabetes-related microvascular complications for patients with T1D. Furthermore, the UK Prospective Diabetes Study (UKPDS) found intensive treatment reduced macrovascular complications for patients with T2D. Informing patients about the relationship between intensive treatment and lessening complications may help motivate patients' active participation. Notably, in a recent study, 62% ($n = 80$) of patients with T1D reported wanting their health-care providers to discuss diabetes complications at diabetes diagnosis or as early as possible in the course of their illness, and many also noted the importance of providers discussing complications with nonblaming explanations, patience, and understanding, as well as specific treatment options to enhance their hope, efficacy, and motivation to improve self-care. Patients sometimes develop negative attitudes about the inevitable development of complications, which may occur when attempts to achieve desired glycemic targets have not succeeded. Success with short-term goals can help alter patient attitudes about the inevitability of complications and may bolster intentions to continue intensive management.

Importantly, diabetes complications also have a significant psychosocial impact on patients' quality of life, with negative outcomes for specific complications such as loss of independence, changes in occupational and family roles, increased social isolation with diabetic retinopathy, psychosocial difficulties with diabetic kidney disease, increased levels of depression, and anxiety in patients with lower-limb amputations. Furthermore, there is a significant and consistent association between depression and retinopathy, nephropathy, neuropathy, sexual dysfunction, and macrovascular complications, as well as an increased prevalence and odds for depression among patients with diabetes and other comorbid chronic diseases.

Complications not only may exact a psychological toll but also may affect a patient's ability to engage in intensive management. Patients may begin to see themselves as handicapped or limited in their ability to carry out an intensive diabetes care regimen once complications are diagnosed. Perceived limitations may be physical or emotional. Onset of complications may be associated with a decline in optimism about treatment efficacy, resulting in less motivation to intensify efforts and reduced quality of life. Education regarding different treatment approaches and supports can renew the patient's commitment to achieving better glycemic control. Patients may need help understanding that any improvement in their glycemic status can improve their overall health status and delay the progression of complications. Health-care professionals also should understand that distressing feelings in response to the diagnosis of complications are an expected and normal response; however, concerns may be warranted if a prolonged emotional response continues to interfere with patient's everyday functioning, and a referral to a mental health professional may be needed.

Coping and Problem-Solving Skills

Coping and problem-solving skills can be taught and practiced. Coping skills involve making prompt and effective changes to the diabetes care regimen when a problem arises. Peyrot and colleagues, in their biopsychosocial model of glycemic control in diabetes, explored the relationships among coping strategies, stress, and diabetes regimen adherence and found that people with T1D who used self-controlled coping (pragmatism and problem-solving) had better glycemic control and diabetes care adherence than those who used emotional coping (anger, impulsive actions, anxious, and avoidant behaviors). Furthermore, a study exploring patient–provider communication found that patients who used more self-controlled coping were less reluctant about discussing their self-care behaviors with providers. Thus, it appears that efforts should be made to promote patients' pragmatic problem-solving approaches to diabetes distress.

Through problem solving, individuals attempt to identify effective and adaptive solutions for specific problems encountered in everyday living. A review of the literature on problem-solving and diabetes found that problem-solving interventions demonstrated improvement in HbA_{1c} for both children and adults and had a positive effect on psychosocial outcomes, such as reduced negative communication between parent and children or adolescents and improved self-efficacy in adults. Effective diabetes-related coping and problem-solving includes

- identifying factors that may contribute to adverse diabetes events (e.g., life stress, comorbidities, changes in insulin or technological devices, routine, eating, or exercise, and alcohol or medication use);
- recognizing one's ability and skills to evaluate the circumstances and respond appropriately; and
- informing and seeking support from a family member or health-care professional who can help problem-solve and collaborate on treatment strategies and behaviors.

DIABETES MANAGEMENT

ADHERENCE SCREENING

Adherence is different than compliance. Rather than simple semantics, the difference implies a philosophy of treatment and expectations of the patients' and health professionals' roles. Compliance assumes an exact prescription for behavior and a hierarchy for treatment, which is counter to a patient-centered approach. With compliance, the provider knows best and the patient must comply with what the provider says without collaborating on the treatment regimen or treatment goals. Adherence assumes patient–clinician collaboration, which includes jointly defining problems, agreeing on specific problems, setting realistic treatment goals, and developing an action plan for achieving goals in the context of patient's life.

Systematic evaluation of adherence is unusual in clinical practice. In most cases, provider evaluation of patient adherence is subjective: partially based on patients' report of what they have or haven't done, reports of adverse events such as hypoglycemia, and more objective data of HbA_{1c} and weight. Interestingly, several studies have shown that some patients report reluctance to discuss their actual self-care behaviors with providers because of shame, guilt, and fear of judgment. Therefore, it is not clear how much health-care professionals actually learn about patients' self-care during treatment encounters. A trusting and nonjudgmental patient–clinician relationship may decrease patients' reluctance to discuss their self-care. Conducting a focused adherence screening in the context of an effective relationship may allow the clinician to assess and develop patients' cooperation and skills so that together they can realistically develop the "best fit" treatment regimen. Some practical steps to engage the patient are listed in Table 4.1.

Table 4.1—Practical Steps to Engage the Patient

Use a questionnaire or an interview to assess the following:

- Gaps in the patient's knowledge of diabetes and skills of diabetes self-care tasks
  - Administer a survey such as Self-Care Inventory-Revised (SCI-R)
- Burden of self-care tasks
  - What is it like to live with these self-care tasks on a daily basis?
- Intentions regarding self-care behaviors
  - How do you intend to change and try this new self-care regimen?
- Attitudes about self-care changes
  - Explain the new self-care regimen. What is not clear?
  - How does the new self-care regimen address your goals for diabetes care?
  - Why or why not will this new self-care regimen have a positive effect on your diabetes?
  - How might this new self-care regimen be too difficult for you to do?
  - How might you be successful with this new self-care regimen?
- Self-efficacy
  - How do you feel ready and able to follow this new self-care regimen?
- Practicing behavior in the following ways:
  - Suggest the patient try a new self-care regimen or new technology
  - Meet more frequently with patient to assess progress with self-care behaviors.

LIFESTYLE CHANGES

Results of the Look AHEAD study and UKPDS have shown us that lifestyle changes, particularly diet and exercise modification, must be implemented in addition to intensified self-care behaviors to achieve optimal metabolic control—especially in patients with T2D. As a result, the role of health-care professionals has expanded to include helping patients initiate and maintain lifestyle changes that support intensive diabetes management. Behavioral strategies are used to achieve these goals within primary care and other medical settings.

Behavioral therapy within a context of social support has been shown to be effective in increasing exercise and modifying dietary intake, resulting in modest weight loss, improved glycemia, and reduced cardiac risk factors. Targeting and monitoring behavior change can be incorporated easily into routine diabetes care. Preliminary discussion of the behavior to be targeted and the goal to be achieved can occur while the physical examination takes place. This allows patients time to reflect on whether they are motivated to tackle changing a behavior at this particular time, consider whether the behavior change is realistic for them, and develop a feasible plan to implement the change. When instituting a behavioral program, the health-care professional may develop an agreement with the patient, which may include the following steps:

1. Identify a behavior that the patient is willing to work to change (e.g., ask "Would you be willing to walk a half hour daily or eat two servings of vegetables daily?"), not one that is "prescribed."
2. Define the behavior in such a way that change can be monitored (e.g., have the patients keep a daily log of the activity).
3. Set a realistic goal for the change that you and the patient agree on (e.g., increase walking from zero times a week to three times a week for a half hour, *not* increase exercise from zero times a week to running 3 miles three times a week).
4. Establish and agree on the methods and supports necessary for the patient to change his or her daily routine (e.g., "What time of day would be convenient for this particular activity?").
5. Set a realistic date to accomplish the goal and for discussing the progress the patient has made using his or her written record.
6. If a routine checkup is not scheduled, arrange to communicate with the patient after 2 weeks regarding his or her progress, successes, and setbacks, during which time the patient and provider can identify barriers to success, generate problem-solving solutions, or modify the goal to make it either more manageable or challenging.
7. At the appointed follow-up visit or through electronic media, assess with the patient whether the new behavior has been mastered or more time is needed to make the behavior routine. If life circumstances have changed, more problem solving may be needed, along with another plan for ensuring maintenance of the new behavior.

Once the agreement is made and documented (including significant others when appropriate), the provider can follow up by phone, fax, e-mail, or in person to monitor the "intervention." Again, if patients are counseled that setbacks and difficulties are expected when changing lifestyle behaviors, a sense of failure can be attenuated if not prevented. Often, small changes in behavior not only improve the patient's medical outcome but also improve quality of life and enhance his or her feelings of efficacy and well-being.

PSYCHOSOCIAL SUPPORT SYSTEM

FAMILY SYSTEM

It is particularly important for the health-care professional to assess the family system regarding attitudes toward intensification and medical care, willingness to participate in diabetes care, and financial resources. Family support is often a critical element in the success of intensive management because family members provide both concrete resources and emotional support for a patient's effort to improve his or her diabetes care. The process of intensifying treatment should be slowed and the health-care professional should consider referral for counseling if family conflict around diabetes management is manifested. It is particularly important for the practitioner to assess the family system regarding attitudes toward intensification and medical care in general, willingness to participate in diabetes care, and financial resources. Conflicts can be avoided by having a clear discussion of diabetes care with all participating family members. This should specify who will take responsibility for which aspects of the regimen, the monitoring functions of each family member, and how the care regimen will or won't affect how the family lives. Attention is warranted when a patient reports being isolated and without a support system. This is especially important for emerging adults who have moved to a new city or for the elderly who live alone.

If motivation and commitment to intensive management come from a parent or a spouse, the relationship needs to be evaluated so that diabetes management does not become a vehicle for family conflict. It may become necessary to refer the patient and family for further diabetes education as well as interpersonal counseling. Family conflict over diabetes management can occur in any family when members disagree about treatment regimens, glycemic goals, and responsibilities of care. Families who are particularly susceptible are those with

- an adolescent patient whose wish for autonomy and independence from parental caretaking results in worsening glycemia;
- young children whose parents do not share the same strategies for self-care or goals;
- family members who perceive and express that the diabetes care routine negatively affects the family environment; or
- family members who feel that their needs are not being met because psychosocial and material resources are disproportionately expended on the family member with diabetes (this may apply to siblings as well as spouses).

Parents increasingly are seeking intensive treatment for their young children and adolescents with T1D or are initiating prevention efforts on behalf of their overweight children or adolescents who have prediabetes. Long-term concerns about the physical well-being of their child place an enormous burden on many parents. Thus, parents may have desires for an intensive treatment regimen that may not be feasible, given the age and maturity of the child. Goals for treatment may not be shared by the child or adolescent and may excessively stress the family system. Issues of autonomy and decision making regarding adherence to the prescribed treatment regimen also can lead to family conflict, regardless of the age of the patient. Decisions about the treatment regimen should be considered in the context of the patient's and family's wishes, adjustment to illness, resources, and abilities of all family members, especially when formulating regimens for children and adolescents. These caveats also apply to spousal systems and adult children taking care of elderly parents with diabetes.

LIVING WITH OTHERS

Interpersonal support often contributes significantly to a patient's ability to implement and maintain intensive management. Psychosocial support can entail emotional support, which is nondirective and supplies a sense of caring and worth; tangible support, which is directive and offers concrete assistance; informational support, which includes guidance and help with problem solving; and companionship support, which offers a sense of social belonging. Psychosocial support can help remove barriers to adherence because it eases the burden of illness; it can come from the whole health-care team, a specific clinician, a family member, a religious leader or organization, or a diabetes support group. Importantly, patients usually are most comfortable seeking support from people and institutions in which they have established trusting relationships. Therefore, long-term continuity of care with health-care professionals is an essential part of intensive management.

A patient's need for support varies depending upon their individual characteristics and social networks. Health-care professionals may facilitate patients seeking support by

- asking patients to identify individuals in their lives who would be willing to be educated to help with intensive diabetes management;
- including significant others in the planning of diabetes care regimens; and
- encouraging patients to share the responsibilities of diabetes care with family and friends to whatever extent they feel comfortable.

In addition, electronic media such as e-mail and text messages can replace phone calls or face-to-face meetings, allowing both patient and health-care professional flexibility and ease of contact. As with other recommendations for care, establish frequency of communication so that expectations are clear between professionals and patients. Additionally, ensure that Health Insurance Portability and Accountability Act regulations are observed and that a clear understanding develops between patient, support personnel, and providers regarding issues of privacy as well as who will be privy to information, particularly if underage children or adolescents are involved or if there are concerns for safety.

Intensified treatment may involve more public exposure of the patient's diabetes. For example, the patient may be less able to retire to a private location to more frequently check blood glucose or give an extra insulin bolus. Thus, intensive treatment may involve a patient coming to terms with the expectations and beliefs of others and needing to become his or her own patient advocate and educator. This may or may not feel comfortable to the individual, and the issue of private versus public business may need to be addressed and practiced. It is a common experience for people with diabetes to be asked, "Are you supposed to be eating that?" or, even more pointedly, to be told they are not supposed to be eating food with sugar. Having planned responses to these comments of "misguided helping" is part of living with diabetes. Anticipating such interactions is part of basic diabetes education, but this topic may need to be revisited during the process of intensification.

PATIENT–HEALTH CARE PROFESSIONAL RELATIONSHIP AND COMMUNICATION

Patient-centered medical treatment promotes physician–patient collaboration. Inherent to this collaboration are physicians' and patients' abilities to communicate effectively, develop a trusting interpersonal relationship, and discuss treatment-related decisions. Patients' active participation in the treatment team is another important part of the patient-centered approach. Patients, however, sometimes are afraid to tell their clinicians that they feel incapable of carrying out the requested behavior, are disinclined to do so because of fear or lack of resources, or disagree with the regimen prescription. Patients who do not feel a rapport with their clinicians are less likely to incorporate and sustain changes to their care regimen. Thus, establishing an atmosphere of collaboration and mutual respect during the treatment encounter will promote patients' cooperation. The collaborative physician–patient relationship in diabetes is associated with increased self-efficacy, improved attitudes toward diabetes and quality of life, decreased negative attitudes toward living with diabetes, and improved glycemic control.

Patients' ability to discuss their self-care successes and difficulties with physicians enables physicians to individualize treatment prescriptions and recommendations, a necessary component of intensified treatment. Furthermore, physicians' ability to openly and effectively respond to patients' self-care reports, discuss immediate and long-term disease concerns, and provide treatment recommendations are important relationship and communication factors for optimal diabetes management. In a study exploring patient and physician perceptions of self-care communication, both physicians and patients recommended trust, nonjudgmental acceptance, open and honest communication, and providing patients hope for living with diabetes as important factors for improving self-care communication. If trusting patient–clinician communication is established, patients may cope more easily with the demands of intensive management.

To promote patient involvement in diabetes management, it is important to

- include patients and their support system in the treatment team;
- collaborate on regimen, treatment goals, and self-care behaviors that are needed to achieve and maintain goals;
- adapt the regimen to the patient's lifestyle;
- have patients practice self-care behaviors;
- monitor the efficacy and outcomes of agreed-upon behaviors and redefine goals as necessary;

- renegotiate the treatment plan or behaviors if the current plan is not working; and, above all,
- stay positive, supportive, and nonjudgmental even when treatment goals are not being met.

HELPING PATIENTS WITH LONG-TERM ADHERENCE

Patient motivation, ability, and intention to maintain a complex regimen will vary over time. Choosing to focus less on diabetes care during periods of emotional turmoil, holidays, and vacation is to be expected. Other life events may temporarily take precedence over intensive diabetes management. By accepting that variation in self-management behaviors is expected (not aberrant), the health-care professional can ensure that periodic lapses do not spiral into a sense of failure and frustration and disengagement from self-care. Some suggestions include the following: *1*) attempt to determine why the lapse in self-care behavior occurred, *2*) enlist the patient in making decisions regarding the redirection of treatment, and *3*) use a collaborative, nonjudgmental approach.

Intensification of diabetes management requires the patient to prioritize the diabetes care regimen. Note that treatment behaviors that have been mutually agreed on may not always result in the expected glycemic outcome. Factors such as stress, other disease processes, or changes in lifestyle or routine may affect glycemic control. Health-care professionals and patients engaged in achieving optimal glycemia should not view unanticipated outcomes as failures of treatment. Instead, patient and clinician can work to identify causal relationships between lifestyle, emotions, and glycemic status to develop self-care coping strategies. Health-care professionals need to help patients understand that unexpected glycemic excursions should not be viewed as a personal failure, poor problem solving, or treatment failure. The connection between new behaviors and glycemic control may not be immediate. Positive regard for small steps in behavior change may provide the support necessary until the patient's behavior becomes self-sustaining.

Helping patients formulate a regimen that is responsive to their lifestyles may ensure greater adherence with the prescribed treatment. A treatment regimen that fits into, rather than controls, lifestyle should be the goal of a maintainable treatment plan. When a patient is resistant to a health-care professional's suggestions, nonadherence should not be assumed. A collaborative dialogue between patient and clinician can reestablish a working plan about self-management wherein the patient agrees to glycemic goals, and together strategies are developed that work toward resumption of intensive glucose goals.

CONCLUSION

Intensive diabetes management is presently the gold standard treatment for most patients with T1D and many patients with T2D who use insulin. Intensive treatment is challenging and patients may burn out, feel distressed, and have difficulties meeting these challenges. Patients also can succeed when they are actively engaged in a collaborative patient–clinician relationship that is part of a multidisciplinary health-care team and are supported psychosocially by family, friends, coworkers, and members of their community. In addition, teaching and promoting patients' coping and problem-solving skills are critically important for improved management of the demanding tasks of intensive treatment as well as life stresses and lifestyle changes.

Active patient engagement requires that clinicians understand and address the psychosocial factors that may promote or interfere with patients' performing or not performing the tasks of intensive diabetes management. Thus, a psychosocial assessment is essential to explore patients' diabetes burnout, diabetes distress, depression, anxiety, eating disorders, and substance abuse, which may serve as barriers to intensive management. When health-care professionals face patients with higher than target HbA_{1c}, they need to stop seeing this simply as nonadherence, but rather should explore the psychosocial factors that may be contributing to patients' difficulties managing their self-care. For example, health-care professionals can begin to consider that the patient's higher A1C may be caused by his or her possible fear of hypoglycemia or an eating disorder involving restricting or omitting insulin, or other psychosocial factors. Through this thoughtful consideration, clinicians may begin to address the underlying psychosocial concerns, and patients may begin to make progress toward achieving their glucose target goals.

Psychosocial assessments should occur both before intensive diabetes management begins and throughout the course of treatment. Once psychosocial concerns have been identified, clinicians need to make appropriate recommendations to address these concerns. This may include referral to a mental health professional who can assess the psychosocial issues contributing to poor glycemia and can use cognitive-behavioral, interpersonal, and family counseling approaches to address the concerns. In addition, the mental health professional needs to be included in the multidisciplinary team, which is integral to the treatment of most psychosocial concerns, particularly eating disorders.

Importantly, patient–clinician collaboration highlights the need for patients' active engagement in treatment. When providers respectfully inquire and listen for potential barriers to intensification, patients are able to set treatment goals that are responsive to their individual lifestyles. This increases the likelihood of successfully achieving these goals and may lessen patients' perceptions of the tasks of intensive treatment as an overwhelming burden.

When patients are diagnosed with both T1D or T2D, they often perceive the specter of diabetes complications in their future. Studies show that patients want to be informed and prepared to address complications as early as possible after diabetes diagnosis and want providers to communicate specific treatment options, demonstrate understanding and patience, and avoid blame. Discussion of the results of the DCCT and more recent studies may act as a motivator for improved glycemia. Patient perception of the inevitability of complications also may impede motivation by fostering negative views and a sense of hopelessness. These views may be enhanced further once complications appear, and the patient's ability and motivation to engage in intensive management may be diminished. At these times, patients would benefit from clinicians engaging in encouraging discussions about how any improvement in their glycemia can improve their overall health status and help delay the progression of complications.

Finally, patients and health-care professionals need to understand and accept that long-term treatment adherence with intensive diabetes management may vary over time. Adherence depends on patients' psychological and physical status and reactions to life events and changes in lifestyle. A supportive treatment team with a trusting patient–health care professional relationship and communication can be a critical underpinning to patients' success in sustaining intensive diabetes management.

BIBLIOGRAPHY

Ahmed AT, Karter AJ, Liu J. Alcohol consumption is inversely associated with adherence to diabetes self-care behaviours. *Diabet Med* 2006;23:795–802

American Diabetes Association. Standards of medical care in diabetes—2015. *Diabetes Care* 2015;38(Suppl. 1):S1–S76

Anderbro T, Gonder-Frederick L, Bolinder J, Lins PE, Wredling R, Moberg E, Lisspers J, Johansson UB. Fear of hypoglycemia: relationship to hypoglycemic risk and psychological factors. *Acta Diabetol* 2015;52:581–589

Anderson RJ, Freedland KE, Clouse RE, Lustman PJ. The prevalence of comorbid depression in adults with diabetes: a meta-analysis. *Diabetes Care* 2001;24:1069–1078

Anderson RJ, Grigsby AB, Freedland KE, de Groot M, McGill JB, Clouse RE, Lustman PJ. Anxiety and poor glycemic control: a meta-analytic review of the literature. *Int J Psychiatry Med* 2002;32:235–247

Beverly EA, Ganda OP, Ritholz MD, Lee Y, Brooks KM, Lewis-Schroeder NF, Hirose M, Weinger K. Look who's (not) talking: diabetes patients' willingness to discuss self-care with physicians. *Diabetes Care* 2012;35:1466–1472

Brod M, Alolga SL, Meneghini L. Barriers to initiating insulin in type 2 diabetes patients: development of a new patient education tool to address myths, misconceptions and clinical realities. *Patient* 2014;7:437–450

Ciechanowski P, Katon WJ. The interpersonal experience of health care through the eyes of patients with diabetes. *Soc Sci Med* 2006;63:3067–3079

Coffey L, Gallagher P, Horgan O, Desmond D, MacLachlan M. Psychosocial adjustment to diabetes-related lower limb amputation. *Diabet Med* 2009;26:1063–1037

DeGroot, M, Anderson R, Freedland KE, Clouse RE, Lustman PJ. Association of depression and diabetes complications: a meta-analysis. *Psychosomat Med* 2001;63:619–630

Diabetes Control and Complications Trial Research Group. The effect of intensive treatment of diabetes on the development and progression of long-term complications in insulin-dependent diabetes mellitus. *N Engl J Med* 1993;329:977–986

DiMatteo, MR. Social support and patient adherence to medical treatment: a meta-analysis. *Health Psychol* 2004;23:207–218

Ducat L, Phillipson LH, Anderson BJ. The mental health comorbidities of diabetes. *JAMA* 2014;312:691–692

Devenney R, O'Neill S. The experience of diabetic retinopathy: a qualitative study. *Br J Health Psychol* 2011;16:707–721

Eaton WW, Armenian H, Gallo J, et al. Depression and outpatient management of eating disorders in type 1 diabetes. *Diabetes Spect* 2009;22:147–152

Egede, LE. Effect of co-morbid chronic diseases on prevalence and odds of depression in adults with diabetes. *Psychosomat Med* 2005;67:46–51

Fisher L, Gonzales JS, Polonsky WH. The confusing tale of depression and distress in patients with diabetes: a call for greater clarity and precision. *Diabet Med* 2014;31:764–772

Fitzpatrick SL, Schumann KP, Hill-Briggs F. Problem solving interventions for diabetes self-management and control: a systematic review of the literature. *Diabetes Res Clin Pract* 2013;100:145–161

Gibbons CH, Freeman R. Treatment-induced neuropathy of diabetes: an acute, iatrogenic complication of diabetes. *Brain* 2015;138(Pt. 1):43–52

Goebel-Fabbri AE, Anderson BJ, Fikkan J, Franko DL, Pearson K, Weinger K. Improvement and emergence of insulin restriction in women with type 1 diabetes. *Diabetes Care* 2011;34:545–550

Goebel-Fabbri AE, Fikkan J, Franko DL, Pearson K, Anderson BJ, Weinger K. Insulin restriction and associated morbidity and mortality in women with type 1 diabetes. *Diabetes Care* 2008;31:415–419

Jones JM, Lawson ML, Daneman D, Olmsted MP, Rodin G. Eating disorders in adolescent females with and without type 1 diabetes: cross sectional study. *BMJ* 2000;320:1563–1566

Kaplan SH, Greenfield S, Ware JE. Assessing the effects of physician-patient interactions on the outcomes of chronic disease. *Med Care* 1988;27:S110–S127

Kenardy J, Mensch M, Bowen K, Green B, Walton J, Dalton M. Disordered eating behaviours in women with type 2 diabetes mellitus. *Eat Behav* 2001;2:183–192

Kroenke K, Spitzer RL, Williams JB. The PHQ-9: validity of a brief depression severity measure. *J Gen Intern Med* 16:606-13, 2001

The Look AHEAD Research Group. Reduction in weight and cardiovascular disease risk factors in individuals with type 2 diabetes: one-year results of the Look AHEAD trial. *Diabetes Care* 2007;30:1374–1383

Lustman PJ, Clouse RE. Treatment of depression in diabetes: impact of mood and medical outcome. *J Psychosomat Res* 2002;53:917–924

Markowitz JT, Butler DA, Volkening LK, Antisdel JE, Anderson BJ, Laffel LM. Brief screening tool for disordered eating in diabetes: internal consistency and external validity in a contemporary sample of pediatric patients with type 1 diabetes. *Diabetes Care* 2010;33:495–500

Nathan DM, Zinman B, Cleary PA, Backlund JYC, Genuth S, Miller R, Orchard TJ. Modern-day clinical course of type 1 diabetes mellitus after 30 years' duration: the Diabetes Control and Complications Trial/Epidemiology of Diabetes Interventions and Complications and Pittsburgh Epidemiology of Diabetes Complications experience (1983–2005). *Arch Intern Med* 2009;169:1307–1316

Peyrot M, McMurry JF, Kruger DF. A biopsychosocial model of glycaemic control in diabetes: stress, coping and regimen adherence. *J Health Soc Behav* 1999;40:141–158

Polonsky WH, Fisher L, Guzman S, Villa-Caballero L, Edelman SV. Psychological insulin resistance in patients with type 2 diabetes: the scope of the problem. *Diabetes Care* 2005;28:2543–2545

Polonsky WH, Fisher L, Earles J, Dudley RJ, Lees J, Mullan JT, Jackson RA. Assessing psychological stress in diabetes. *Diabetes Care* 2005;28:626–631

Polonsky WH, Anderson BJ, Lohrer PA, Aponte JE, Jacobson AM, Cole CF. Insulin omission in women with IDDM. *Diabetes Care* 1994;17:1178–1785

Radloff LS. The CES-D scale: a self-report depression scale for research in the general population. *Appl Psychol Meas* 1977;1:385–401

Ritholz M, MacNeil T, Vangala D, Weinger K. Patients' responses to initial diagnosis of diabetes complications. *Diabetes* 2015;64(Suppl. 1):A230

Ritholz MD, Beverly EA, Brooks KM, Abrahamson MJ, Weinger K. Barriers and facilitators to self-care communication during medical appointments in the United States for adults with type 2 diabetes. *Chronic Illn* 2014;10:303–313

Ritholz MD, Beste M, Edwards, SS, Beverly EA, Atakov-Castillo, A, Wolpert, HA. Impact of continuous glucose monitoring on diabetes management and marital relationships of adults with type 1 diabetes and their spouses: a qualitative study. *Diabet Med* 2014;31:47–54

Rubin RR, Peyrot M. Psychological issues and treatments for people with diabetes. *J Clin Psychol* 2001;57:457–478

Stetson B, Schlundt D, Peyrot M, Ciechanowski P, Austin M, Young-Hyman D, McKoy J, Hall M, Dorsey R, Fitzner K, Quintana M, Narva A, Urbanski P, Homko C, Sherr D. Monitoring in diabetes self-management: issues and recommendations for improvement. *Popul Health Manag* 2011;14:189–197

Strom JL, Egede LE. The impact of social support on outcomes in adult patients with type 2 diabetes: a systematic review. *Curr Diab Rep* 2012;12:769–781

Surwit RS, Schneider MS, Feinglos MN. Stress and diabetes mellitus. *Diabetes Care* 1992;15:1413–1422

Tamborlane WV, Beck RW, Bode BW, Buckingham B, Chase HP, Clemons R, et al. Continuous glucose monitoring and intensive treatment of type 1 diabetes. *N Engl J Med* 2008;359:1464–1476

TODAY Study Group, Wilfley D, Berkowitz R, Goebel-Fabbri A, Hirst K, Ievers-Landis C, Lipman TH, Marcus M, Ng D, Pham T, Saletsky R, Schanuel J, Van Buren D. Binge eating, mood, and quality of life in youth with type 2 diabetes: baseline data from the TODAY Study. *Diabetes Care* 2011;34:858–860

UK Prospective Diabetes Study Group. Intensive blood glucose control with sulfonylurea or insulin compared with conventional treatment and risks of complications in patients with type 2 diabetes (UKPDS 33). *Lancet* 1998;352:837–853

Von Korff M, Gruman J, Schaefer J, Curry SJ, Wagner EH. Collaborative management of chronic illness. *Ann Intern Med* 1997;127:1097–1102

Weinger K, Butler HA, Welch GW, La Greca AM. Measuring diabetes self-care: a psychometric analysis of the Self-Care Inventory-Revised with adults. *Diabetes Care* 2005;28:1346–1352

Weitzman ER, Ziemnik RE, Huang Q, Levy S. Alcohol and marijuana use and treatment nonadherence among medically vulnerable youth. *Pediatrics* 31 August 2015 [Epub ahead of print]

Welch GW, Jacobson AM, Polonsky WH. The Problem Areas in Diabetes scale: an evaluation of its clinical utility. *Diabetes Care* 1997;20:760–766

Zuijdwijk CS, Pardy SA, Dowden JJ, Dominic AM, Bridger T, Newhook LA. The mSCOFF for screening disordered eating in pediatric type 1 diabetes. *Diabetes Care* 2014;37:e26–e27

Patient Selection, Clinical Considerations, and Intensive Diabetes Management Goals

DOI: 10.2337/9781580406321.05

Highlights
Patient Selection, Clinical Considerations, and Intensive Diabetes Management Goals

- Appropriate patient selection is important in individualizing the right treatment regimen and set of treatment goals.
- Patient characteristics that influence intensive diabetes management include
  - desire to improve glycemic management;
  - willingness to be actively involved in care;
  - access to adequate diabetes education;
  - ongoing, open communication with health-care team; and
  - presence of adequate support networks.
- A successful treatment regimen is one that can be adapted to meet lifestyle needs, balances the patient's risks and benefits, and is subject to ongoing evaluation and modification.
- No one set of glycemic goals can be applied to every person with diabetes. Glycemic targets must be modified according to the patient's age, disease duration, type of diabetes, prior hypoglycemia history, lifestyle, diabetes complications status, concurrent medical conditions, and support network.
- If intensive diabetes management is deemed inadvisable for a particular patient, efforts must be made to encourage whatever degree of glycemic improvement is individually and safely possible.

Patient Selection, Clinical Considerations, and Intensive Diabetes Management Goals

Successful intensive diabetes management must incorporate diabetes self-management principles and strategies. The relative effectiveness of intensive management efforts is influenced by individual patient characteristics as well as the efforts of his or her health-care team. In the past two decades basal-bolus insulin replacement regimens have become the mainstay of intensive diabetes treatment, and the question should not be about selecting the "right patient" but rather about how best to engage patients who might have a harder time reaching the recommended targets or for whom intensive management may be contraindicated. These concepts will be the primary focus of this chapter.

GLYCEMIC GOALS OF INTENSIVE MANAGEMENT

Appropriate patient selection is crucial to support the pursuit of glycemic targets that are as close to normal as safely possible for each individual (see Table 5.1). Tar-

Table 5.1 — Guidelines for Intensive Management Targets

Nonpregnant adults

Glycated hemoglobin A$_{1c}$	<7%*
Preprandial capillary plasma glucose	80–130 mg/dL (4.4–7.2 mmol/L)**
Peak postprandial capillary plasma glucose	<180 mg/dL (<10.0 mmol/L)

Postprandial glucose should be targeted if A1C goals are not met despite achievement of preprandial glucose goals.
More stringent glycemic goals (i.e., <6.0%) may further reduce complications at the cost of increased risk of hypoglycemia.

Conception and pregnancy

Preprandial capillary blood glucose	≤90 mg/dL (5.0 mmol/L)
and either:	
1-h postprandial capillary blood glucose	≤130–140 mg/dL (7.2–7.8 mmol/L)
or	
2-h postprandial capillary blood glucose	≤120 mg/dL (6.7 mmol/L)

*Referenced to a nondiabetic range of 4.0–6.0% using a DCCT-based assay.
**Postprandial glucose measurements should be performed 1–2 h after the beginning of the meal.

get ranges for preprandial, postprandial, and bedtime glycemia serve as the reference goal for most patients with diabetes. These targets, however, do not incorporate assessment of overnight blood glucose levels to mitigate the risk of nocturnal hypoglycemia. Most of the severe hypoglycemic episodes in the Diabetes Control and Complications Trial (DCCT) occurred nocturnally (43%) or during sleep (55%) and, accordingly, the overnight blood glucose goals often need to be higher.

CLINICAL CONSIDERATIONS

Goals of intensive diabetes management should be individualized using a collaborative process with the patient and the health-care team (see Table 5.2). All patients should be encouraged and supported to reach the most intensified glucose goals they are capable of achieving.

If the patient's choice is based on knowledge of what intensive management would entail, the patient's treatment choice should be accepted by the health-care team. The clinician should try to present a balanced review of perceived benefits and risks and avoid being judgmental or critical toward the patient's decision. Motivation to improve diabetes self-management cannot be forced. Health-care professionals can help by noticing, acknowledging, and encouraging even small, positive changes and to continue to assess readiness to make larger changes over time. Ongoing communication and education about diabetes management options, their benefits and risks, and an understanding of specific patient concerns may encourage patients to move toward more intensified management over time.

Health-care professionals need to be sensitive to potential barriers in meeting the rigorous demands of an intensive diabetes regimen. The patient's age and interpersonal support, as well as intellectual, emotional, financial, occupational, and domestic status, need to be taken into account when customizing an intensive treatment regimen and defining glycemic targets.

- Is the patient cognitively and emotionally capable of assuming primary responsibility for daily care and treatment decisions?
- If not, is there a responsible individual who is willing to be educated and to actively participate in this complex regimen?
- If the patient lives alone, who will have daily or frequent contact with the patient in case of emergencies, such as severe hypoglycemia or illness requiring outside intervention?

Table 5.2—Patient Characteristics to Consider in Intensive Diabetes Management

- Desire to improve glycemia
- Willingness to become actively involved in daily management
- Skill in diabetes self-management techniques
- Awareness and acceptance of benefits and risks associated with intensive management
- Ongoing, open, and honest communication with health-care team
- Family or personal support

- Does the patient's home, work, or academic environment permit and support the behaviors needed for intensive treatment?
- Does the patient have the financial resources to pay for the increased costs associated with intensive treatment (e.g., more frequent visits for medical care, education and counseling, blood glucose monitoring, supplies, and equipment)?

A collaborative relationship between the patient and health-care team is most likely to lead to an effective management plan that is tailored to the individual. Such a regimen must be adaptable to meet the individual's lifestyle needs, must carefully balance the risks and benefits of therapy, and must be evaluated and modified over time. This means the patient must be willing and ideally want to have regular contact with the health-care team. Through this frequent contact, effective changes can be made and problem-solving skills can be developed and reinforced. This process is facilitated and strengthened when the patient feels that he or she is valued as an equal team member and sees that the team is interested in his or her own ideas and provides him or her with the sense of being accepted and supported rather than judged or blamed when struggling. When the health-care relationship is built on those characteristics, intensive management efforts have the potential to enhance flexibility, improve quality of life, and promote a sense of improved mastery over diabetes.

Intensive diabetes management should be considered for most individuals with type 1 diabetes (T1D). Indeed, it is the current and standard medical treatment for the disease. Implementation is strongly recommended for

- motivated individuals, with no early evidence of complications;
- women who are pregnant or contemplating pregnancy; and
- individuals with newly diagnosed diabetes.

Caution and care should be exercised when determining whether to pursue intensive treatment for specific subsets of the population with T1D and type 2 diabetes (T2D; see Table 5.3). All treatment decisions must weigh the benefits of the treatment against its associated risks.

PATIENTS WITH TYPE 2 DIABETES

Intensive diabetes management should also be considered for most individuals with T2D. Although treatments for T2D differ from those for T1D, frequent blood glucose monitoring, nutrition management, physical activity, and ongoing communication with the health-care team are crucial components of the treatment regimen for both forms of the disease. Lowering pre- and postprandial blood glucose toward the normal range is desirable, especially in those with shorter duration of diabetes or absence of cardiovascular disease. If this can be accomplished by regimens involving nutritional counseling, physical activity, healthy weight loss, oral or injected glucose-lowering agents, or simple insulin regimens (e.g., intermediate-acting insulin, premixed insulin once or twice a day, or a long-acting insulin once daily), then a more intensive insulin regimen may not be necessary. Treatment options that are weight neutral or that have modest associated weight loss should be

Table 5.3—Patient Characteristics That May Influence the Treatment Goals and Feasibility of Intensive Management of Diabetes

- Hypoglycemia unawareness
- A history of recurrent severe hypoglycemic episodes
- Use of medications that may interfere with hypoglycemia detection or treatment (e.g., ß-blockers)
- Other medical conditions that can be aggravated by hypoglycemia (e.g., cerebrovascular disease or angina)
- Severe psychiatric disorders, impaired cognitive ability, or psychosocial stressors
- Alcohol or drug abuse problems
- Advanced end-stage diabetes complications
- Cardiovascular disease and longer duration type 2 diabetes
- Symptomatic coronary artery disease
- Cardiac arrhythmias
- Concurrent diseases or conditions that would functionally limit intensive management (e.g., debilitating arthritis or severe visual impairment)
- Relatively short life expectancy/elderly patients
- Age <6 years

considered first. As the disease progresses, many patients will benefit from intensive insulin regimens. The goals of therapy may require further modification because of hypoglycemia or additional weight gain.

The patient and medical characteristics listed in Tables 5.2 and 5.3 should be considered for patients with both T1D and T2D. Many of the characteristics listed in Table 5.3 relate to patient difficulties with hypoglycemia, especially hypoglycemia unawareness. Hypoglycemia unawareness previously was considered to be an absolute contraindication to adoption of an intensive treatment regimen. This is no longer the case and, in fact, the tools used in intensive diabetes management (i.e., insulin pumps and continuous glucose monitors) can be of benefit in reducing risk for hypoglycemia associated with tight glycemic control. In addition, in most patients, unawareness can be reversed by meticulous avoidance of hypoglycemia for ~2–4 weeks.

When practicing intensive management, some episodes of mild hypoglycemia are expected and considered acceptable, as long as they are well recognized, appropriately treated, and do not interfere with day-to-day life. Mild hypoglycemia becomes unacceptable when the safety of patients or those around them is placed at risk. For example, even mild hypoglycemia needs to be avoided during the operation of a motor vehicle or complex machinery. Patients for whom it is determined that risky behavior or faulty decision making are contributing to frequent episodes of hypoglycemia should be referred for behavioral evaluation or intervention. In most cases, strategies that significantly reduce risk can be created jointly. If a patient persists in risk-taking, then the health-care team needs to strongly urge the patient to consider altering glycemic targets, which may require involving significant others in monitoring activities. Some factors to consider when establishing treatment goals are listed in Table 5.4.

Table 5.4—Factors to Consider When Establishing Individualized Treatment Goals

- Age
- Ability of patient to understand and implement a complex treatment regimen
- Disease duration
- Type of diabetes (type 1, type 2, or gestational)
- History of repeated, severe hypoglycemia
- Ability to recognize hypoglycemic symptoms
- Lifestyle and occupation (e.g., possible risks of experiencing hypoglycemia on the job)
- Presence and severity of diabetes complications
- Presence of other medical conditions or treatments that might alter the response to therapy or prevent the patient from carrying out self-care behaviors
- Financial constraints
- Level of support available from family and friends

GOAL-SETTING FOR SPECIAL POPULATIONS

No single set of blood glucose targets can be applied to every person with diabetes. What might be recommended for an otherwise healthy young adult with T1D early in the course of the illness may differ markedly from what is recommended for an older adult with T2D and coronary artery disease and reduced vision or for a toddler with working parents who spends most of the day in a day-care setting. Factors that play a role in determining the glycemic goals for any patient include age, ability to assume responsibility for decision making, duration of diabetes, type of diabetes, prior history of hypoglycemia, lifestyle or occupation, presence or absence of complications, other medical conditions or treatments, and availability of support from family or friends (Table 5.4).

CULTURE

Patients' beliefs about health, illness, and provider–patient roles often are embedded in their cultures. Therefore, before beginning intensive management, cultural factors need to be considered and openly discussed, especially because diabetes is prevalent among such diverse cultural groups. If health-care providers are not aware of or do not consider patients' cultural beliefs, then treatment goals and prescriptions may go unheeded and nonadherence may be misunderstood. The following example from Asian American culture highlights health-care providers' needs to learn about, be aware of, and thoughtfully incorporate patients' cultural beliefs and practices with intensive management. A cross-sectional survey of 9,187 adults representative of the California population found that nearly three-quarters of the Asian Americans assessed used at least one type of traditional Chinese medicine in the past 12 months. Again, providers' sensitivity to the diverse cultures represented by their patients and an interest in learning about their potential impact on health-care practices and understanding can increase adherence with diabetes management.

PREGNANCY

A lower glycemic target range is recommended during pregnancy to improve outcomes. The American Diabetes Association (ADA) recommends preprandial glucose levels ≤90 mg/dL (5.0 mmol/L) and either 1-h postprandial levels of 130–140 mg/dL (7.2–7.8 mmol/L) or 2-h postprandial levels of ≤120 mg/dL (6.7 mmol/L). Accomplishment of these targets requires more effort on the part of the patient and the health-care team as well as frequent communication and active support. Avoidance of recurrent or severe hypoglycemia must be considered in the pursuit of these stringent glycemic goals.

CHILDREN

Children, especially those <6–7 years old, require a team with special expertise and experience in the management of childhood diabetes. When such a team is available, intensive diabetes management is encouraged.

The patient's history of severe hypoglycemia and associated neurological and neuropsychological risk needs to be carefully considered when setting individualized glycemic targets for children with T1D. Children <6–7 years old are particularly vulnerable to the long-term adverse effects of severe or repeated hypoglycemia. For young children with a developing central nervous system, significant hypoglycemia may be associated with loss of cognitive function that may be transient or permanent. We also know that hypoglycemia interferes with information processing, and repeated hypoglycemia may disrupt academic progress. Therefore, the avoidance of hypoglycemia is an especially important goal in this age-group, resulting in glycemic targets that are higher than targets in older children and adults. For children <6 years old, the ADA recommends preprandial glucose levels of 100–180 mg/dL (5.6–10 mmol/L) and bedtime or overnight values of 110–200 mg/dL (6.1–11.1 mmol/L). When a child can reliably report symptoms of hypoglycemia and obtain or carry out prompt treatment, premeal glycemic targets can be lowered to 80–170 mg/dL (4.4–9.4 mmol/L).

Premeal glucose values of 90–180 mg/dL (5.0–10.0 mmol/L) and values of 100–180 mg/dL (5.6–10.0 mmol/L) at bedtime or overnight are recommended for school-age children (6–12 years of age). For adolescents and young adults (13–19 years of age), premeal glucose values of 90–130 mg/dL (5.0–7.2 mmol/L) and bedtime or overnight values of 90–150 mg/dL (5.0–8.3 mmol/L) are recommended. Postprandial blood glucose testing is indicated in situations in which a discrepancy is noted between the premeal blood glucose values and A1C and to better assess overall glycemia. When individualizing the glycemic goals, always consider the risks versus benefits, and the capabilities and wishes of the family as well as the child.

OLDER ADULT PATIENTS

Goals for therapy in older adult patients warrant special consideration. When treating older adults (>65 years old), setting treatment goals and targets may be complicated because of coexisting chronic conditions, such as cognitive dysfunction, depression, and physical disabilities as well as polypharmacy. These issues may interfere with patients' abilities to perform self-care tasks, such as glucose monitoring, following complex insulin regimens, and adhering to recommended diet and exercise. In addition, older adults are often reluctant to make changes in their insulin doses between clinic visits or during illnesses. In older and frail patients, the focus in treatment often needs to be on avoiding malnutrition and hypoglycemia rather than strict glycemic control. Less-stringent A1C goals (such as 8%) may be appropriate for patients with a history of severe hypoglycemia, risk of falling, advanced microvascular or macrovascular complications, extensive comorbid conditions, and limited life expectancy. Assessing the individual's specific health characteristics and resources should inform the establishment of appropriate glycemic targets to avoid increasing risk.

CONCLUSION

Achieving lower glycemic targets for all individuals with diabetes is the goal of intensive treatment. The relationship between glycemia and long-term complications must be considered in the context of the cost-to-benefit ratio associated with this treatment. If treatment strategies are to be effective in reducing long-term sequelae, then treatment goals and implementation techniques must be maintainable over time. Not all patients will be able to cope with the demands of intensive diabetes management, but most patients will benefit from improvements in glucose control. Failure to achieve glycemic targets should signal the need to reevaluate self-care behaviors and possibly to tailor intervention strategies. Ongoing encouragement and support for achieving even small but medically meaningful improvements is crucial. Inability to reach the ideal glycemic target must not be viewed as a treatment failure or a patient failure.

No patient should be dismissed arbitrarily as ineligible or unsuitable for intensified diabetes management efforts. Instead, each patient should be evaluated critically for his or her ability and willingness to use intensive diabetes management, given the requisite knowledge, skills, and resources. The health-care professional is uniquely positioned to monitor, guide, encourage, and collaborate with the patient in the pursuit of long-term health.

BIBLIOGRAPHY

American Association of Diabetes Educators (AADE). *The Art and Science of Diabetes Self-Management Education.* Chicago, AADE, 2006

American Diabetes Association. Standards of medical care in diabetes—2016. *Diabetes Care* 2016;39(Suppl. 1):S1–S111

American Diabetes Association. *Medical Management of Type 1 Diabetes.* 5th ed. Kaufman F, Ed. Alexandria, VA, American Diabetes Association, 2008

American Diabetes Association. *Medical Management of Type 2 Diabetes.* 6th ed. Burant C, Ed. Alexandria, VA, American Diabetes Association, 2008

Cryer PE. Hypoglycaemia: the limiting factor in the glycaemic management of type I and type II diabetes. *Diabetologia* 2002;45:937–948

Cryer PE, David SN, Shamoon H. Hypoglycemia in diabetes. *Diabetes Care* 2003;26:1902–1912

Diabetes Control and Complications Trial–Epidemiology of Diabetes Interventions and Complications (DCCT–EDIC) Research Group. Retinopathy and nephropathy in patients with type 1 diabetes four years after a trial of intensive therapy. *N Engl J Med* 2000;342:381–389

Holman RR, Paul SK, Bethel MA, Matthews DR, Neil HA. 10-year follow-up of intensive glucose control in type 2 diabetes. *N Engl J Med* 2008;359:1577–1589

Hsiao AF, Wong MD, Goldstein MS, Becerra LS, Cheng EM, Wenger NS. Complementary and alternative medicine use among Asian-American subgroups: prevalence, predictors, and lack of relationship to acculturation and access to conventional health care. *J Compl Alt Med* 2006;12:1003–1010

Jacobson AM, Musen G, Ryan CM, Silvers N, Cleary P, Waberski B, Burwood A, Weinger K, Bayless M, Dahms W, Harth J; the DCCT/EDIC Research Group. Long-term effect of diabetes and its treatment on cognitive function. *N Engl J Med* 2007;356:1842–1852

Jacobson AM, Ryan CM, Cleary PA, Waberski BH, Weinger K, Musen G, Dahms W; the DCCT/EDIC Research Group. Biomedical risk factors for decreased cognitive functioning in type 1 diabetes: an 18-year follow-up of the DCCT cohort. *Diabetologia* 2011;54:245–255

Juvenile Diabetes Research Foundation Continuous Glucose Monitoring Study Group. Factors predictive of use and of benefit from continuous glucose monitoring in type 1 diabetes. *Diabetes Care* 2009;32:1947–1953

Kitzmiller JL, Block JM, Brown FM, Catalano PM, Conway DL, Coustan DR, Gunderson EP, Herman WH, Hoffman LD, Inturrisi M, Jovanovic LB, Kjos SI, Knopp RH, Montoro MN, Ogata ES, Paramsothy P, Reader DM, Rossen BM, Thomas AM, Kirkman MS. Managing pre-existing diabetes in pregnancy: summary of evidence and consensus recommendations for care. *Diabetes Care* 2008;31:1060–1079

Look AHEAD Research Group. Reduction in weight and cardiovascular disease risk factors in individuals with type 2 diabetes: one-year results of the Look AHEAD trial. *Diabetes Care* 2007;30:1374–1783

Martin CL, Albers J, Herman WH, Cleary P, Waberski B, Greene DA, Stevens MJ, Feldman EL. Neuropathy among the Diabetes Control and Complications Trial cohort 8 years after trial completion. *Diabetes Care* 2006;29:340–344

Metzger BE, Buchanan TA, Coustan DR, de Leiva A, Dunger DB, Hadden DR, Hod M, Kitzmiller JL, Kjos SL, Oats JN, Pettitt DJ, Sacks DA, Zoupas C. Summary and recommendations of the Fifth International Workshop-Conference on Gestational Diabetes Mellitus. *Diabetes Care* 2007;30(Suppl. 2):S251–S260

Munshi MN, Segal Ar, Suhl E, Ryan C, Sternthal A, Giusti J, Lee Y, Fitzgerald S, et al. Assessment of barriers to improve diabetes management in older adults a randomized controlled study. *Diabetes Care* 2013;36:543–549

Nathan DM, Cleary PA, Backlund JY, Genuth SM, Lachin JM, Orchard TJ, Raskin P, Zinman B. Intensive diabetes treatment and cardiovascular disease in patients with type 1 diabetes. *N Engl J Med* 2005;353:2643–2653

Nathan DM, Zinman B, Cleary PA, Backlund JYC, Genuth S, Miller R, Orchard TJ. Modern-day clinical course of type 1 diabetes mellitus after 30 years' duration: the Diabetes Control and Complications Trial/Epidemiology of Diabetes Interventions and Complications and Pittsburgh Epidemiology of Diabetes Complications experience (1983–2005). *Archives of Internal Medicine* 2009;169:1307–1316

Nathan DM, Buse JB, Davidson MB, Ferrannini E, Holman RR, Sherwin R, Zinman B. Medical management of hyperglycemia in type 2 diabetes: a consensus algorithm for the initiation and adjustment of therapy—a consensus statement of the American Diabetes Association and the European Association for the Study of Diabetes. *Diabetes Care* 2009;32:193–203

Perranti DC, Lima A, Wu J, Weaver P, Warren SL, Sadler M, White NH, Hershey T. Effects of prior hypoglycemia and hyperglycemia on cognition in children with type 1 diabetes mellitus. *Pediatr Diabetes* 2008;9:87–95

Peranti DC, Wu J, Koller JM, Lim A, Warren SL, Black KJ, Sadler M, White NH, Hershey T. Regional brain volume differences associated with hyperglycemia and severe hypoglycemia in youth with type 1 diabetes. *Diabetes Care* 2007;30:2331–2337

Silverstein J, Klingensmith G, Copeland KC, Plotnick L, Kaufman F, Laffel L, Deeb LC, Grey M, Anderson BJ, Holzmeister LA, Clark NG. Care of children and adolescents with type 1 diabetes mellitus: a statement of the American Diabetes Association. *Diabetes Care* 2005;28:186–212

Skyler JS, Bergenstal R, Bonow RO, Buse J, Deedwania P, Gale EA, Howard BV, Kirkman MS, Kosiborod M, Reaven P, Sherwin RS, American Diabetes Association, American College of Cardiology Foundation, American Heart Association. Intensive glycemic control and the prevention of cardiovascular events: implications of the ACCORD, ADVANCE, and VA diabetes trials: a position statement of the American Diabetes Association and a scientific statement of the American College of Cardiology Foundation and the American Heart Association. *Diabetes Care* 2009;32:187–192

Stratton IM, Adler AI, Neil HA, Matthews DR, Manley SE, Cull CA, Hadden D, Turner RC, Holman RR. Association of glycaemia with macrovascular and microvascular complications of type 2 diabetes (UKPDS 35): prospective observational study. *BMJ* 2000;321:405–412

UK Prospective Diabetes Study Group. Intensive blood glucose control with sulfonylureas or insulin compared with conventional treatment and risk of complications in patients with type 2 diabetes. *Lancet* 1998;352:837–853

Weber P, Weberova D, Meluzinova H. How to approach to the therapy of diabetes in the elderly. *Adv Gerontol* 2014;27:519–530

Whitmer RA, Karter AJ, Yaffe K, Quesenberry CP Jr, Selby JV. Hypoglycemic episodes and risk of dementia in older patients with type 2 diabetes mellitus. *JAMA* 2009;301:1565–1572

Wolpert HA, Anderson BJ. Metabolic control matters: why is the message lost in translation? The need for realistic goal-setting in diabetes care. *Diabetes Care* 2001;24:1301–1303

Multicomponent Insulin Regimens

DOI: 10.2337/9781580406321.06

Highlights
Multicomponent Insulin Regimens

- Multicomponent insulin regimens use four types of insulin:
  - The human insulin analogs lispro, aspart, and glulisine have the most rapid onset of action and time to peak effect and the shortest duration.
  - The intermediate-acting insulin (NPH insulin; also called isophane) has a more delayed onset of action and peak effect and a longer duration of action.
  - The analog insulins U-100 glargine and detemir have relatively long action profiles and are nearly peakless.
  - New analog insulin degludec recently was approved, which has even longer action profiles than glargine and detemir and is peakless.
- Insulin absorption and availability are influenced by
  - anatomical regions of injections, with the fastest absorption from the abdomen and the slowest from the thigh;
  - timing of premeal injections;
  - factors such as exercise, showering, bathing, and ambient temperature; and
  - injection of insulin into areas of lipoatrophy, scarring, and lipohypertrophy.
- Multicomponent insulin regimens attempt to mimic physiological insulin release.
  - These regimens consist of various conformations of basal and prandial insulin components.
  - Frequent self-monitoring of blood glucose (SMBG) guides appropriate changes in insulin dosage and timing, food intake, and activity profile.
  - Prandial insulin is administered by syringe, pen, or insulin pump.
  - Basal insulin is administered with a rapid-acting analog by insulin pump or by injection of NPH, glargine, detemir, or degludec.
- Specific insulin regimens allow individual, flexible combinations of insulins and analogs that are suitable for various lifestyles, including
  - premeal regular or rapid-acting (lispro, aspart, glulisine) insulin and basal glargine, detemir, or degludec;
  - premeal regular or rapid-acting (lispro, aspart, or glulisine) basal NPH; and
  - continuous subcutaneous insulin infusion of rapid-acting or regular insulin.

- Other insulin programs that offer less flexibility and generally less intensive management options are
  - twice-daily mixtures of regular or rapid-acting insulin and NPH;
  - prebreakfast rapid-acting insulin or regular insulin and NPH, predinner rapid-acting or regular insulin, and bedtime NPH; and
  - prebreakfast rapid-acting or regular insulin, predinner rapid-acting or regular insulin, and glargine, detemir, or degludec in the morning, evening, or both.
- Initial insulin dosages usually range from 0.2 to 1.0 units/kg body wt/day. Dosage requirements vary considerably during the remission or "honeymoon" phase (when there is residual β-cell function), intercurrent illness, adolescence, or pregnancy.
- Insulin dosage is then divided into basal and prandial injections:
  - Forty to fifty percent provides basal insulin.
  - The remainder is divided among the meals, using insulin-to-carbohydrate ratios or preset dose guidelines.
  - All regimens must be individualized to the patient's desires, lifestyle, age, comorbidities, concomitant medications, and defined target level of glycemic control.
- Insulin adjustments consist of an action plan for the alteration of therapy to achieve individually defined glycemic goals.
  - Changes are made in insulin dosage, timing of injections, or the meal plan guided by SMBG results.
  - Pattern adjustments consist of modification in the current insulin dosage to minimize glycemic excursions throughout the day and to avoid hypoglycemia (<70 mg/dL).

Multicomponent Insulin Regimens

This chapter discusses the design and use of insulin regimens for intensive diabetes management.

INSULIN PHARMACOLOGY

INSULIN TIMING AND ACTION

There are five general categories of time course of insulin action:

- rapid-acting insulin (e.g., insulin lispro, aspart, and glulisine [genetically engineered insulin analogs]);
- short-acting insulin (e.g., regular [soluble]);
- intermediate-acting insulin (NPH, isophane);
- long-acting insulin (glargine and detemir [genetically engineered insulin analogs]); and
- ultralong-acting insulin (degludec [genetically engineered insulin analog]).

Table 6.1 summarizes the nominal action profiles—time to peak action and duration of action—of these insulin preparations.

Two general pharmacokinetic principles apply: First, a longer time to peak results in a broader peak and longer duration of action. Second, with increasing insulin dose, the breadth of the peak and the duration of action tend to be somewhat lengthened. The values included in Table 6.1 are for doses of 10–15 units, or 0.1–0.2 units/kg.

Rapid-Acting Insulin

Three genetically engineered insulin analogs designed to have a rapid onset and short duration of action when injected subcutaneously are currently available. Insulin lispro, [Lys(B28), Pro(B29)]-human insulin, contains an inversion of the amino acids at positions 28 and 29 of the B-chain. Insulin aspart, [Asp(B28)]-human insulin, contains a substitution of the proline at position 28 of the B-chain with aspartate. Insulin glulisine contains a lysine at B3 replacing asparagine, and a glutamic acid at B29 replaces lysine. These analogs have similar pharmacokinetic properties. They are sterile, aqueous, clear, and colorless, and they have a neutral pH. In contrast to native human insulin, the modifications in the insulin molecule

Table 6.1—Insulins by Comparative Action

	Onset	Peak Action	Effective Duration
Rapid acting			
Insulin lispro (analog)*	5–15 min	30–90 min	3–5 h
Insulin aspart (analog)*	5–15 min	30–90 min	3–5 h
Insulin glulisine (analog)	5–15 min	30–90 min	3–5 h
Short acting			
Regular (soluble)	30–60 min	2–3 h	5–8 h
Intermediate acting			
NPH (isophane)	2–4 h	4–10 h	10–16 h
Long acting			
Insulin glargine (analog)	2–4 h	Peakless	20–24 h
Insulin detemir (analog)	2–4 h	6–14 h	16–20 h
Ultralong acting			
Insulin degludec (analog)	30–90 min	Peakless	24–42 h
Combinations			
70% NPH, 30% regular	30–60 min	Dual	12–18 h
70% NPA, 30% aspart	5–15 min	Dual	12–18 h
75% NPL, 25% lispro	5–15 min	Dual	12–18 h
50% NPL, 50% lispro	5–15 min	Dual	12–18 h

*Per manufacturers' data; other data indicate equivalent pharmacodynamic effect.
Source: Plank J, Wutte A, Brunner G, Siebenhofer A, Semlitsch B, Sommer R, Hirschberger S, Pieber TR. Direct comparison of insulin aspart and insulin lispro in patients with type 1 diabetes. *Diabetes Care* 25:2053–2057.

inhibit its ability to self-aggregate into hexamers and dimers in solution. This enables insulin to be more rapidly absorbed from the subcutaneous tissue after injection.

Short-Acting Insulin

Regular (soluble or unmodified) insulin has the most rapid onset and shortest duration of action of any native insulin preparation (i.e., human insulin that is not modified to change its pharmacokinetic properties) with an onset at 30–60 min, a peak effect 2–3 h after administration, and an effective duration of action of 3–6 h. Because of interindividual variation, in some patients, an effect is evident for up to 8 h. Duration of action may be longer with large doses or when patients have insulin antibodies.

Intermediate-Acting Insulin

NPH insulin, which is an intermediate-acting insulin, uses protamine to retard and extend insulin action. The addition of protamine creates an insulin suspension, and after injection, insulin is more slowly absorbed from the subcutaneous tissue. NPH insulin has an onset of action 2–4 h after injection, a peak effect 4–10 h after administration, and an effective duration of action of 10–16 h.

Long-Acting Insulin

U-100 Insulin glargine. U-100 insulin glargine is a genetically modified insulin analog (21A-Gly-30Ba-L-Arg-30Bb-L-Arg-human insulin). The amino acid asparagine at position A21 is replaced by glycine, and two arginines are added to the C-terminus of the B-chain. The effect of these changes is to shift the isoelectric point, producing a solution that is completely soluble at pH 4. When injected into the subcutaneous tissue, which has a physiological pH of 7.4, the acidic solution is neutralized. This leads to the formation of microprecipitates, or stabilized aggregates, from which small amounts of insulin glargine are slowly released. Glargine is absorbed from abdominal subcutaneous injection sites at a relatively constant rate, with no prominent peak in serum insulin concentration for 24 h.

Insulin detemir. Insulin detemir is a long-acting basal insulin analog with a duration of action up to 24 h. Insulin detemir differs from human insulin in that threonine has been omitted from position B30 and a C14 fatty acid chain has been attached to the amino acid at position B29. Insulin detemir is a clear, colorless, aqueous neutral sterile solution at pH 7.4. Its prolonged action is the result of slow systemic absorption of insulin detemir molecules from the injection site caused by strong self-association of the molecules and binding to albumin. Insulin detemir is more slowly distributed to peripheral target tissues because it is highly bound to albumin in the bloodstream. Compared with NPH, both insulin glargine and insulin detemir have less dose-to-dose variability in pharmacodynamics.

Ultralong-Acting Insulin

Insulin degludec (*INN/USAN*) is an ultralong-acting insulin analog. It has one single amino acid deleted in comparison to human insulin and is conjugated to hexadecanedioic acid via γ-L-glutamyl spacer at the amino acid *lysine* at position B29. The addition of hexadecanedioic acid to lysine at the B29 position allows for the formation of multihexamers in subcutaneous tissue, or subcutaneous depot, that results in slow insulin release into the systemic circulation. The onset of action is 30–90 min, and its duration of action is up to 42 h. Because of its ultralong action, it can be given at any time of the day every day.

Compared with U-100 glargine insulin, degludec has lower incidence of nocturnal hypoglycemia in both T2D and T1D because of its low day-to-day variability. It can be used at the same unit dose as the total daily long- or intermediate-acting insulin unit dose. The safety and efficacy in children and adolescents <18 years old has not been established. Insulin degludec also has the ability to be mixed with short-acting insulin aspart.

Insulin Mixtures

There are commercially prepared, stable mixtures of regular and NPH insulins, insulin lispro protamine suspension (NPL) and insulin lispro, and insulin aspart protamine suspension (NPA) and insulin aspart. These mixtures contain either 70% NPH and 30% regular insulin or 70% NPA and 30% insulin aspart (called "70/30"), and 75% NPL and 25% lispro (called "75/25"). These premixed insulins may be helpful in elderly patients, blind patients, patients with cognitive impairment, or other patients who have difficulty mixing insulin in a syringe or using complex insulin regimens. These mixtures limit flexible dosing, however, and necessitate that the patient be on a fixed meal plan.

A newly approved mixture with ultralong-acting insulin degludec and insulin aspart (IDegAsp; Ryzodeg) consists of 70% ultralong-acting basal insulin (IDeg) and 30% rapid-acting insulin (IAsp IDegAsp). This insulin formulation can be given once a day using a dose corresponding to 70% of total daily dose, with the remaining 30% split and given as insulin aspart at the other meals.

Concentrated Formulations of Insulin

In recent years, several more concentrated formulations of insulin have become available. These formulations have the same amount of units in smaller volume (i.e., U-200 has 200 units insulin in 1 mL, U-300 has 300 units in 1 mL) and are available in pens that display the number of units. The dose dialed into the pen by the patient is the dose dispensed by the device. In contrast, with U-500 insulin, which is available in a vial, the insulin needs to be administered with a syringe (or pump), which needs to be considered when drawing up insulin doses. To avoid dosing errors, it can be safer to dispense U-500 insulin using Tuberculin syringes, rather than insulin syringes (with the Tuberculin syringe, every 0.1 mL will contain 50 units of insulin).

STABILITY OF INSULINS

Because insulin is stable for long periods when refrigerated, it should be stored in a refrigerator. Insulin, however, is generally stable at room temperature for 28 days and does not need to be stored in the refrigerator after the bottle is opened, as long as it is used within this time. In contrast, insulin should not be exposed to extreme temperatures (e.g., in the car, near a window, or by a heating or air conditioning vent). It should not be exposed to direct sunlight or heat (including temperatures $\geq 30°C$ [$\geq 86°F$]) and should not be frozen.

Regular insulin and the synthetic insulin analogs (lispro, aspart, glulisine, detemir, glargine, and degludec) are all in solution. All other insulin preparations are in suspension. Vials containing NPH, NPL, and NPA insulin suspensions must be gently rolled at least 10 times (it has been recommended that pens containing NPH insulin be rolled and tipped 20 times) to ensure uniform suspension before insulin is withdrawn from the vial.

On mixing insulins, physiochemical changes may occur (either immediately or over time). As a result, the physiological response to the insulin mixture may differ from that of the insulins injected separately. Mixtures of two types of insulin vary in stability. Regular, lispro, aspart, glulisine, and NPH-type insulins are freely miscible in all proportions. These insulins may be mixed in the same syringe and their action profiles may be maintained. A decrease in the absorption rate (but not total bioavailability) is seen when insulin lispro, aspart, or glulisine is mixed with NPH insulin. Most or all of the rapid action of regular insulin or the rapid-acting analogs is retained, however, if mixing is done in a syringe immediately before injection. The acidic nature of insulin glargine precludes its mixture with other insulins. Also, insulin detemir should not be mixed with any other insulins because it can substantially reduce their absorption profile. The acidic nature of insulin glargine precludes its mixture with other insulins.

INSULIN ABSORPTION

Many factors influence insulin absorption and alter insulin availability. Intra-individual variation in insulin absorption from day to day can vary by as much as ⁻25%, and between patients, by up to 50%. The newer longer-acting insulin ana-logs—such as degludec, determir, and both glargine formulations—have less dose-to-dose variability in pharmacodynamics than the older intermediate-acting insulin such as NPH. In general, as the dose is increased, the absorption of subcu-taneously injected insulin becomes more prolonged.

Injection Site

Insulin absorption differs across injection sites, especially for short-acting insulins (regular, lispro, aspart, and glulisine). Absorption is most rapid from the abdomen, followed by the arm, buttocks, and thigh. These differences are the likely the result of variation in blood flow. The variation is sufficiently great that random rotation of injection sites should be avoided, if possible. Patients should rotate injection sites within regions, rather than between regions, for any given injection, to decrease day-to-day variability. Because insulin absorption is most rapid in the abdomen (in the absence of exercise), it may be the preferred site for preprandial injections. Some patients use the abdomen for all preprandial injec-tions, whereas others use the abdomen for the prebreakfast injection and other regions for prelunch or predinner injections.

Timing of Premeal Injections

Timing of preprandial insulin injections is crucial to matching insulin action with carbohydrate absorption. Insulin lispro, glulisine, and aspart have a rapid onset of action and generally should be given ~15 min before starting to eat a meal. With more rapidly absorbed high-glycemic-index carbohydrate meals, it sometimes can be necessary to bolus even earlier to provide appropriate coverage for the meal. Conversely, early administration of insulin before meals containing more slowly digested lower glycemic index carbohydrates, such as pasta, can result in early postprandial hypoglycemia, and in these situations, insulin often is best given immediately before the meal. In practice, review of continuous glucose trac-ings can be informative in defining optimal bolus timing for specific meals. Sub-cutaneous regular insulin should be injected at least 20–30 min before eating a meal. The timing of injections also should be altered depending on premeal gly-cemia. When blood glucose levels are above a patient's target range, the interval between insulin administration and meal consumption should be increased to per-mit the insulin to lower blood glucose toward the target range. For example, when the premeal glucose is above target, rapid-acting insulin can be given 15–30 min and regular insulin 30–60 min before the meal. If premeal blood glucose levels are below a patient's target range, regular insulin should be injected immediately before meal consumption. Rapid-acting insulin analog administration should be delayed until after the patient has consumed carbohydrates and the blood glucose level has been restored to normal. In certain circumstances (if the ability of the patient to consume the meal is uncertain), it is prudent to wait until immediately after completing the meal to administer rapid-acting insulin. The presence of gastroparesis diabeticorum may significantly delay carbohydrate absorption. In these patients, postmeal insulin administration or the use of regular insulin, which has a longer onset of action, may be advantageous.

Factors Influencing Insulin Absorption

Physical exercise increases blood flow to an exercising body part and accelerates absorption of insulin from that region. Sporadic exercise may induce variability in insulin absorption. The patient should avoid injections in a body region that will be exercised while that injection is being absorbed. For example, if the patient intends to jog shortly after an injection, he or she should avoid giving that injection into the thigh. When exercise is contemplated, the patient might use the abdomen preferentially, because this region is the least likely to have significant increases in absorption (unless sit-ups are planned). Other factors influencing absorption of regular insulin are ambient temperature (e.g., a hot bath or sauna), smoking, and local massage of the injection site.

Thin patients with little subcutaneous tissue face an increased risk of intramuscular rather than subcutaneous injection, which leads to more rapid absorption of any given insulin preparation. This risk can be averted by using short needles. Also, the interval between injection of preprandial regular insulin and meal consumption may need to be shortened. Some parents have reported that in thin, young children, insulin analogs are best administered immediately after a meal is eaten, both because of the rapid onset and the ability to ensure that the child has eaten before insulin administration.

INSULIN REGIMENS

MULTICOMPONENT INSULIN REGIMENS: GENERAL POINTS

There are two components of physiological insulin secretion: continuous basal insulin secretion and incremental prandial insulin secretion (see Fig. 6.1). Basal insulin secretion restrains hepatic glucose production, keeping it in equilibrium with basal glucose use by the brain and other tissues that are obligate glucose consumers. After meals, prandial insulin secretion stimulates glucose use and storage while inhibiting hepatic glucose output, thereby limiting the meal-related glucose excursion. Patients with type 1 diabetes (T1D) lack both basal and prandial insulin secretion. Thus, insulin programs for T1D require multiple components that mimic physiological insulin secretion by providing basal insulin and prandial insulin coinciding with each meal. Normal physiological insulin requirements include administration of a background of basal insulin secretion given between meals and overnight. This insulin should be combined with boluses of insulin that coincide with the rise in glucose that accompanies food ingestion with meals and large snacks. The most flexible regimens used for intensive diabetes management

- emphasize the need for preprandial insulin before each meal, separate from basal insulin;
- allow liberal food choices in terms of size, timing, and potential omission of meals while still balancing food intake with activity and insulin dosage; and
- include frequent monitoring of therapy to promote a more normal lifestyle.

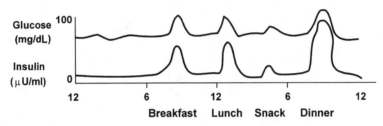

Figure 6.1—Schematic representation of 24-h plasma glucose and insulin profiles in a hypothetical individual without diabetes.

Instrumental to the overall plan is self-monitoring of blood glucose (SMBG) multiple times daily. The patient takes action based on the SMBG results, which are used to help make appropriate changes in insulin dosage and timing, carbohydrate intake, and physical activity. The changes are made according to a predetermined plan provided by the health-care team to the patient.

Prandial Insulin Therapy

Prandial incremental insulin secretion is best duplicated by giving preprandial injections of a rapid-acting insulin analog (lispro, aspart, or glulisine) before each meal by syringe, pen, or pump. Each preprandial insulin dose is adjusted individually to provide insulin appropriate to the current blood glucose level and the meal. If exercise is planned after the meal, insulin doses may need to reduced accordingly. Recent data indicate that dietary fat and protein can affect mealtime insulin requirements (see Chapter 9, Nutrition Management), and insulin doses may need to be adjusted. Regular insulin often will provide more optimal coverage of higher-fat foods such as pizza.

Basal Insulin Therapy

Basal insulin is given as

- one or two daily injections of long-acting insulin (U-100 glargine or detemir) or ultralong-acting insulin (degludec or U-300 glargine),
- intermediate-acting insulin (NPH) at bedtime and as a small morning dose, or
- the basal component of a continuous subcutaneous insulin infusion (CSII) program.

SPECIFIC FLEXIBLE MULTICOMPONENT INSULIN REGIMENS

Premeal Rapid- and Basal Long-Acting Insulins

A premeal program uses three preprandial insulin injections of a rapid-acting insulin (lispro, aspart, or glulisine) and long-acting degludec or glargine (Fig. 6.2) or detemir (Fig. 6.3) insulin to provide basal insulin. If given twice a day, insulin detemir is a relatively peakless insulin. Glargine is also peakless in most patients when given once a day, and it reaches a steady state 3–5 h after administration.

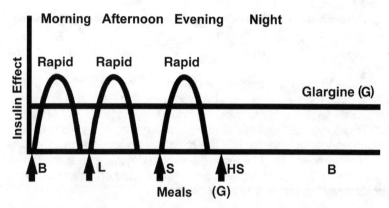

Figure 6.2—Schematic representation of idealized insulin effect by multiple-dose regimen providing basal long-acting insulin glargine (G)and preprandial injections of rapid-acting insulin. Symbols: B, breakfast; L, lunch; S, dinner; HS, bedtime. Arrows indicate time of insulin injection. Although frequently given at HS, the basal insulin may be given at other times of the day and may be required twice a day.

Insulin degludec is relatively peakless after injection and has a sustained duration of action of >42 h. Because it lasts >24 h, the low day-to-day variation in its glucose-lowering effect allows patients who forget a dose, or who for other reasons cannot administer their scheduled dose, greater flexibility in dosing time.

U-100 insulin glargine has a broad peak 15–18 h after injection and a sustained action of 18–24 h. It is sufficiently peakless to provide adequate daily basal insulin. If given with dinner, the waning effect after 18–20 h may result in late afternoon hyperglycemia; therefore, bedtime administration may provide better coverage. For children who require snacks for adequate caloric intake, the addition of a small amount of NPH in the morning may obviate the need for administration of rapid-acting insulin at snack time. For young children who require little basal insulin between 4:00 and 7:00 A.M., morning administration may be optimal.

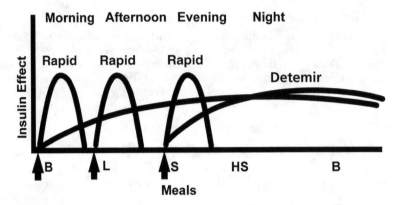

Figure 6.3—Schematic representation of idealized insulin effect by multiple-dose regimen providing basal long-acting detemir insulin and preprandial injections of rapid-acting insulin. Symbols: B, breakfast; L, lunch; S, dinner; HS, bedtime. Arrows indicate time of insulin injection. Although frequently given at HS, the basal insulin may be given at other times of the day and may be required twice a day. Whatever the time of day that the basal insulin is given, it is best injected on a regular schedule approximately the same time each day.

Insulin detemir has a broad peak ~6–8 h after injection and, when given twice a day, may have sustained action up to 24 h. In most patients, twice-daily detemir at steady state has such a sufficiently blunted peak that it behaves like a peakless basal insulin. As a consequence of the waning insulin effect after 20–24 h, if detemir insulin is administered as a single morning dose, glucose levels may increase before the next injection. Thus, it is best to divide detemir insulin into two doses. In practice, detemir can optimize glucose control in individuals who have different day versus night basal requirements and in those who want the flexibility to adjust basal insulin (analogous to the use of the pump temporary basal feature to compensate for increased activity).

Premeal Rapid- and Basal Intermediate-Acting Insulins

This older premeal regimen, which is less commonly prescribed in the 21st century, uses three prandial insulin injections (lispro, glulisine, or aspart) and intermediate-acting insulin (NPH) given at bedtime to provide overnight basal insulin with peak serum insulin levels before breakfast (a time of a relative increase in insulin requirements because of insulin resistance known as the "dawn phenomenon"; see Fig. 6.4). Bedtime administration of intermediate-acting insulin also reduces the risk of nocturnal hypoglycemia. A small morning dose of intermediate-acting insulin (perhaps 20–30% of the bedtime dose) provides daytime basal insulin.

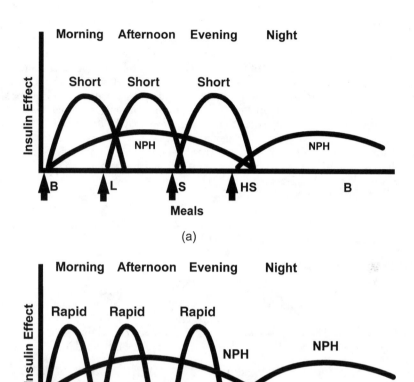

Figure 6.4—Schematic representation of idealized insulin effect by multiple-dose regimens providing basal intermediate-acting insulin at bedtime and before breakfast and preprandial injections of short- (a) or rapid- (b) acting insulin. Symbols: B, breakfast; L, lunch; S, dinner; HS, bedtime. Arrows indicate time of insulin injection.

The basal-bolus regimen has become increasingly popular in recent years for a variety of reasons. It offers flexibility in meal size and timing if the dose is adjusted. (If a preset dose is taken, the same amount of carbohydrates should be consumed.) This regimen is straightforward and easy to understand and implement, because each meal and each period of the day has a well-defined insulin component providing primary insulin action. If snacks containing >15–20 g of carbohydrate are required, as in the growing child or the pregnant patient, additional doses of rapid-acting insulin are required for these snacks.

CSII

The most accurate way to mimic normal insulin secretion clinically is to use an insulin pump in a program of CSII (see Fig. 6.5). The CSII pump continually delivers rapid-acting insulin analog (lispro, aspart, glulisine), thus replicating basal insulin secretion. Moreover, to optimize glycemia, the basal rate may be programmed to vary at times of diurnal variation in insulin sensitivity that adversely affect glycemic control. Thus, the basal infusion rate may be decreased overnight to avert nocturnal hypoglycemia or may be increased to counteract the dawn phenomenon, which often results in hyperglycemia on waking. Temporary basal rates may be used and different patterns may be established, corresponding to the needs of shift workers or people with differing amounts of physical activity on given days. For more on CSII, see Chapter 7.

INSULIN DOSE AND DISTRIBUTION

INITIAL INSULIN DOSES

In typical patients with T1D who are within 20% of their ideal body weight, in the absence of an intercurrent infection or other cause of metabolic instability, the total daily insulin dose required for glycemic control is usually 0.3–1.0 units/ kg body wt/day. The dose is lower during the remission or honeymoon period early in the course of the disease (e.g., 0.2–0.6 units/kg body wt/day). Moreover,

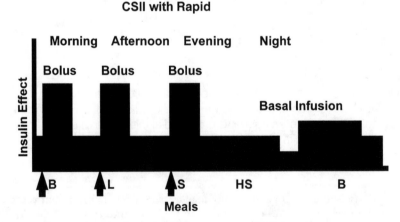

Figure 6.5—Schematic representation of idealized insulin effect provided by CSII of rapid-acting insulin. Symbols: B, breakfast; L, lunch; S, dinner; HS, bedtime. Arrows indicate time of premeal insulin bolus.

during the remission or honeymoon period, as a result of some continuing endogenous insulin secretion, it may be relatively easy to achieve near-normal glycemic control with virtually any insulin program.

During intercurrent illness, the insulin requirements may increase markedly (even doubling). Doses (in units per kilogram) progressively increase during pregnancy. Because the patient's weight also increases, the total dose may even triple. Insulin requirements typically increase throughout puberty and may reach 1.3–1.5 units/kg body wt/day, during the adolescent growth spurt.

INSULIN DOSE DISTRIBUTION

In general, ~40–50% of the total daily insulin dose is used to provide basal insulin. The remainder is divided among the meals, primarily proportionate to the carbohydrate content of the meals. As a starting point, when optimizing prandial insulin dosing, bolus doses are calculated based on the number of grams of carbohydrate consumed. Ultimately, the goal is for the patient to be able to match the meal boluses to the intake of carbohydrate at each meal and snack with an individualized ratio of 1 unit of insulin per specific amount of carbohydrate. This is called the insulin-to-carbohydrate ratio. In practice, it is useful to ask the patient to follow a prescribed meal plan based on the patient's usual dietary intake to establish the patient's insulin-to-carbohydrate ratio. In children, the ratio of insulin to carbohydrate depends on age, body size, pubertal status, and activity level, with a range of ~0.3–1.0 units for every 10 g of carbohydrate consumed. The insulin-to-carbohydrate ratio should be individualized through the use of dietary intake records and blood glucose responses. Breakfast generally requires a slightly larger amount of insulin per gram of carbohydrate and there may be individual reasons for differences at other times of day as well. Alternatively, a constant carbohydrate diet can be prescribed with a fixed insulin dose based on the prescribed carbohydrate content (see Chapter 9). Some patients desire or require a dose of rapid-acting insulin to cover a bedtime snack.

INSULIN ADJUSTMENTS

Patients are provided with an action plan to alter their therapy to achieve individual, defined blood glucose targets before and after meals, at bedtime, and overnight. These actions are guided by SMBG determinations and daily records. Actions may include changing the timing of insulin injections in relation to meals, changing the amount or content of food to be consumed, or altering insulin doses.

Two general types of adjustments are used: acute (usually preprandial) adjustments and pattern adjustments. The acute adjustments (also called corrective doses) provide an action plan that permits immediate action to be taken in response to current circumstances. Pattern adjustments provide an action plan that permits corrective action to be taken when a recurrent pattern is seen in blood glucose fluctuations. Attainment of therapeutic goals requires that both types of adjustments be used.

ACUTE ADJUSTMENTS

Acute adjustments may include changes in food intake and in timing of insulin administration as well as changes in insulin dosage. In practice, most patients find adjustments in the insulin dose to be the most convenient adjustment to make. For especially low blood glucose values, however, additional carbohydrate is urgently needed, and for exceptionally high blood glucose values, a delay in the meal after the insulin dose may be needed. Many experts avoid the term "sliding scale," because the traditional sliding scale did not recognize ongoing (basal and prandial) insulin requirements and would prescribe no insulin when the blood glucose level was in the target range.

Acute adjustments are intended to correct momentary deviations of blood glucose outside the target range and frequently are referred to as "correction doses." The correction may be used when the person experiences a variation in activity, intercurrent illness, or other stress or needs to correct variations in glycemia. The correction dose is in addition to the usual prandial and basal doses.

Corrections actually may be decrements (negative corrections, e.g., lowering of preprandial insulin in anticipation of postprandial exercise or in the face of prevailing blood glucose levels lower than the preprandial target). For patients on a constant carbohydrate diet, corrections (positive or negative) may be given for a larger or smaller carbohydrate meal.

Preprandial corrections provide an action plan for the patient guided by SMBG determinations and daily records. Calculations for corrective insulin dose are given in Chapter 7. One method of calculating the "correction factor" (i.e., the amount of additional insulin needed with a meal to restore the blood glucose to the target level) is to use the "rule of 1,500 or 1,800"—that is, 1,500 or 1,800 divided by the total daily dose of insulin is used to estimate the effect of rapid-acting insulin on the blood glucose level. Thus, in a patient with a blood glucose level of 250 mg/dL and an insulin sensitivity factor of 1 unit per 50 mg/dL, the correction dose would be 3 units of rapid-acting insulin for a target glucose of 100 mg/dL. Obese patients with type 2 diabetes (T2D) typically are insulin resistant and require a higher correction dose, as calculated by the previous formula.

Dosing decision making will depend on the answers to several questions that the patient asks at the time of any premeal insulin injection:

- What is my blood glucose now?
- What do I plan to eat now (i.e., how much carbohydrate and fat will I consume)?
- Do I plan to have an alcoholic beverage with the meal?
- What do I plan to do after eating (i.e., usual activity, increased activity, or decreased activity)?
- What did I do in the past hour (i.e., usual activity, increased activity, or decreased activity)?
- What has happened under these circumstances previously?

The answers to these questions dictate the treatment response and become sensible routine decisions. The usual intervention is an adjustment in the insulin dose, but alterations in food intake (altering the amount or content of food), activity, and timing of injections in relation to meals also may be used.

Table 6.2—Glucose Pattern Analysis Plan

This plan assumes that the preprandial and bedtime blood glucose target is 80–130 mg/dL. Plans should be individualized for each patient.
Insulin assumptions

- Basal insulin (bedtime NPH, glargine, or detemir) is the major insulin acting overnight. Its effect is reflected in the results of blood glucose measurements during the middle of the night and on arising the next morning.
- Basal insulin (morning NPH, bedtime glargine, or bedtime or morning detemir) is the insulin acting and affecting glucose levels when meals are skipped and, in the later morning and later afternoon (i.e., >4 h after the premeal insulin dose).
- Prebreakfast rapid-acting insulin (lispro, aspart, or glulisine) has major action after breakfast. Its effect is primarily reflected in the results of blood glucose measurements 2–3 h after breakfast.
- Prelunch rapid-acting insulin (lispro, aspart, or glulisine) has major action after lunch. Its effect is primarily reflected in the results of blood glucose measurements 2–3 h after lunch.
- Predinner rapid-acting insulin (lispro, aspart, or glulisine) has major action between dinner and bedtime. Its effect is primarily reflected in the results of blood glucose tests 2–3 h after dinner.

If postprandial testing is not being performed, a pattern of rising PREMEAL and HS BG throughout the day with overnight correction may reflect excessive basal insulin relative to prandial insulin, with insufficiency of prandial dosing. This pattern often can be inferred without having many results of 2–3 hr postprandial testing.

PATTERN ADJUSTMENTS

Pattern analysis allows for adjustment in the insulin dose when the blood glucose is consistently above or below the target range at a particular time of day. When a pattern is identified, action should be taken to correct the high or low blood glucose at that time of day (see Table 6.2). The insulin dose (of the relevant insulin component most likely responsible) must be either increased or decreased to correct the pattern of glycemia outside the target range. Pattern analysis with insulin dose adjustments allows prospective changes to be made based on analysis of retrospective data. Pattern analysis can be especially effective when continuous glucose monitoring (CGM) is used, either retrospectively to evaluate diurnal changes in glucose levels, or prospectively to aid the patient to make dose adjustments. These adjustments do not depend on the blood glucose at the moment when they are implemented. Instead, they anticipate the insulin need for the future.

INJECTION DEVICES

Making insulin injections easier and more comfortable enables patients to comply with a treatment plan. In particular, patients may be more willing to initiate intensive diabetes management if a multiple daily insulin injection regimen is made more convenient. Examples of injection devices include insulin pens and an injection port.

Insulin pens are especially useful in intensive insulin therapy. Insulin cartridges containing units of regular, lispro, aspart, glulisine, NPH, 75/25, 50/50, or 70/30 insulin are placed in a pen-like device. Prefilled disposable pens are also available. Disposable needles (variable lengths available) are attached to the end of the insulin pen. The desired dose is administered by turning a dial selector, plunging the needle into the subcutaneous tissue, and pushing a button at the end of the insulin pen to inject the insulin. Insulin pens are convenient to carry in a pocket, purse, backpack, or briefcase and make insulin injections easy to administer away from the home. They eliminate the need to draw up insulin frequently throughout the day.

An injection port includes small needles or Teflon catheters with an external port that can be inserted into subcutaneous tissue of the abdomen or other sites and remain in place for several days. Injections can be given through the catheter instead of through the skin, thus reducing the number of needle punctures.

CONCLUSION

Intensive diabetes management involves flexible multicomponent insulin regimens tailored to the lifestyle of the patient. These regimens distinguish between basal insulin and preprandial insulin, using separate insulin components for different times of the day. Therapy is guided by frequent SMBG, at least four times daily. Patients follow action plans that guide them in daily self-management—altering insulin doses and timing, food intake, or activity—to achieve the selected target level of glycemia. Patient education, collaboration, and motivation are critical to successful program implementation.

BIBLIOGRAPHY

American Diabetes Association, *Practical Insulin: A Handbook for Providers*. 4th ed. Alexandria, VA, American Diabetes Association, 2015

Apidra [packet insert]. Bridgewater, NJ, Sanofi-Aventis U.S. LLC, 2008

Beaser RS, Blair E, Cooppan R. Using insulin to treat diabetes—general principles. In *Joslin's Diabetes Deskbook, A Guide for Primary Care Providers*. 2nd ed. Beaser RS, Ed. Philadelphia, Lippincott Williams & Wilkins, 2007, p. 249–279

Becker RHA. Insulin glulisine complementing basal insulins: a review of structure and activity. *Diabetes Technol Therap* 2007;9:109–121

Bolli GB. Physiological insulin replacement in type 1 diabetes mellitus. *Exp Clin Endocrinol Diabetes* 2001;109(Suppl. 2):S317–S332

Cheng AYY, Zinman B. Principles of insulin therapy. In *Joslin's Diabetes Mellitus* 14th ed. Kahn CR, Weir GC, Eds. Philadelphia, Lippincott Williams & Wilkins, 2005, p. 659–670

Colombel A, Murat A, Krempf M, Kuchly-Anton B, Charbonnel B. Improvement of blood glucose control in type 1 diabetic patients treated with lispro and multiple NPH injections. *Diabet Med* 1999;16:319–324

Danne T, Deiss D, Hopfenmuller W, Von Schutz W, Kordonouri O. Experience with insulin analogues in children. *Horm Res* 2002;57(Suppl. 1):46–53

Davidson J. Strategies for improving glycemic control: effective use of glucose monitoring. *Am J Med* 2005;118(Suppl. 9A):27s–32s

Del Prato S. In search of normoglycaemia in diabetes: controlling postprandial glucose. *Int J Obes Relat Metab Disord* 2002;26(Suppl. 3):S9–S17

Diabetes Control and Complications Trial (DCCT) Research Group. Implementation of treatment protocols in the Diabetes Control and Complications Trial. *Diabetes Care* 1995;18:361–375

Dornhorst A, Luddeke H-J, Sreenan S, Koenen C, Hansen JB, Tsur A, Landstedt-Hallin L. Safety and efficacy of insulin detemir in clinical practice: 14-week follow up data from type 1 and type 2 diabetes patients in the PREDICTIVE™ European cohort. *Int J Clin Pract* 2007;61:523–528

Frid A, Hirsch L, Gaspar R, Hicks D, Kreugel G, et al. New injection recommendations for patients with diabetes. *Diabetes Metab* 2010;36:S3–S18

Gong WC. Determining effective insulin analog therapy based on the individualized needs of patients with type 2 diabetes mellitus. *Pharmacotherapy* 2008;28:1299–1308

Grey M, Boland EA, Tamborlane WV. Use of lispro insulin and quality of life in adolescents on intensive therapy. *Diabetes Educ* 1999;25:934–941

Hanefeld M, Temelkova-Kurktschiev T. Control of post-prandial hyperglycemia—an essential part of good diabetes treatment and prevention of cardiovascular complications. *Nutr Metab Cardiovasc Dis* 2002;12:98–107

Heise T, Heinemann L: Rapid and long-acting analogues as an approach to improve insulin therapy: an evidence-based medicine assessment. *Curr Pharm Des* 2001;7:1303–1325

Heller S, Buse J, Fisher M, Garg S, Marre M, Merker L, Renard E, Russell-Jones D, Philotheou A, Ocampo Francisco A, Pei H, Bode B, on behalf of the BEGIN Basal-Bolus Type 1 Trial Investigators. Insulin degludec, an ultra-longacting basal insulin, versus insulin glargine in basal-bolus treatment with mealtime insulin aspart in type 1 diabetes (BEGIN Basal-Bolus Type 1): a phase 3, randomised, open-label, treat-to-target non-inferiority trial. *Lancet* 2012;379:1489–1497

Hirsch IB, Bode B, Courreges JP, Dykiel P, Franek E, Hermansen K, King A, Mersebach H, Davies M. Insulin degludec/insulin aspart administered once daily at any meal, with insulin aspart at other meals versus a standard basal-bolus regimen in patients with type 1 diabetes: a 26-week, phase 3, randomized, open-label, treat-to-target trial. *Diabetes Care* 2012;35:2174–2181

Hirsch IB. Clinical review: realistic expectations and practical use of continuous glucose monitoring for the endocrinologist. *J Clin Endocrinol Metab* 2009;94:2232–2238

Hofman PE, Derrak JBG, Pinto TE, Tregurtha A, et al. Defining the ideal injection techniques when using 5-mm needles in children and adults. *Diabetes Care* 2010;32:1940–1944

Hoogma RPLM, Schumicki D. Safety of insulin glulisine when given by continuous subcutaneous infusion using an external pump in patients with type 1 diabetes. *Horm Metab Res* 2006;38:429–433

Kovatchev BP, Cox DJ, Gonder-Frederick L, Clarke WL. Methods for quantifying self-monitoring blood glucose profiles exemplified by an examination of blood glucose patterns in patients with type 1 and type 2 diabetes. *Diabetes Technol Ther* 2002;4:295–303

Levemir [packet insert]. Princeton, NJ, NovoNordisk Inc., 2007

Mudaliar S, Edelman SV. Insulin therapy in type 2 diabetes. *Endocrinol Metab Clin North Am* 2001;30:935–982

Peyrot M, Rubin RR, Kruger DF, Travis LB. Correlates of insulin injection omission. *Diabetes Care* 2010;33:240–245

Ratner RE, Hirsch IB, Neifing JL, Garg SK, Mecca TE, Wilson CA, U.S. Study Group of Insulin Glargine in Type 1 Diabetes. Less hypoglycemia with insulin glargine in intensive insulin therapy for type 1 diabetes. *Diabetes Care* 2000;23:639–643

Rosenstock J, Davies M, Home PD, Larsen J, Koenen C, Schernthaner G. A randomized, 52-week, treat-to-target trial comparing insulin detemir with insulin glargine when administered as add-on to glucose-lowering drugs in insulin-naïve people with type 2 diabetes. *Diabetologia* 2008;51:408–416

Rosenstock J, Park G, Zimmerman J, U.S. Insulin Glargine (HOE 901) Type 1 Diabetes Investigator Group. Basal insulin glargine (HOE 901) versus NPH insulin in patients with type 1 diabetes on multiple daily insulin regimens. *Diabetes Care* 2000;23:1127–1142

Ruben RR, Peyrot M, Kruger DF, Travis LB. Barriers to insulin injection therapy. *Diabetes Educ* 2009;35:1014–1022

Skyler JS. Insulin treatment. In *Therapy for Diabetes Mellitus and Related Disorders*. 5th ed. Lebovitz HE, Ed. Alexandria, VA, American Diabetes Association, 2009, p. 207–223

Tsui E, Barnie A, Ross S, Parkes R, Zinman B. Intensive insulin therapy with insulin lispro: a randomized trial of continuous subcutaneous insulin infusion versus multiple daily insulin injection. *Diabetes Care* 2001;24:1722–1727

Vajo Z, Duckworth WC. Genetically engineered insulin analogs: diabetes in the new millennium. *Pharmacol Rev* 2000;52:1–9

Diabetes Technology: Insulin Infusion Pump Therapy and Continuous Glucose Montoring

DOI: 10.2337/9781580406321.07

Highlights
Diabetes Technology: Insulin Infusion Pump Therapy and Continuous Glucose Monitoring

- Insulin therapy by an insulin infusion pump approximates physiological insulin delivery by continuously delivering a basal rate of short- or rapid-acting insulin and allowing bolus insulin administration before meals.

- For the motivated and capable patient with the necessary resources, insulin pump therapy is indicated for
  - suboptimal glycemic control;
  - wide blood glucose excursions;
  - dawn phenomenon with elevated fasting blood glucose levels;
  - nocturnal hypoglycemia;
  - frequent severe hypoglycemia;
  - pregnancy or planned pregnancy;
  - gastroparesis;
  - day-to-day variations in schedule that are not well managed by multiple insulin injections; or
  - patient preference for more flexibility.

- The basal rate should consist of 40–60% of the patient's total daily insulin dose. Several different basal rates can be set in a 24-h period to accommodate diurnal variations in insulin sensitivity.

- Meal boluses are calculated based on carbohydrate content, using an individual ratio of 1 unit of insulin per a specific number of grams of carbohydrate, usually 1 unit of insulin for every 10–20 g carbohydrate for adults and, for example, 1 unit of insulin for every 20–30 g carbohydrate for children or insulin-sensitive adults.

- The patient's insulin sensitivity factor (ISF) or correction factor, which describes the effect of 1 unit of insulin on a patient's blood glucose level, is used to compute the correction dose of insulin that will bring premeal or between-meal hyperglycemia to glycemic target range. The ISF is individualized and is calculated using a formula. An alternative to calculating the ISF is to initiate an ISF of 50 mg/dL for adults and 75–100 mg/dL for children or insulin-sensitive adults.

- Patients can be taught to make additional adjustments in the basal rate or bolus size for illness, exercise, and menses.

- Risks of insulin pump therapy include
    - skin infections, which can be avoided or resolved with regular changes of the infusion set, by keeping the infusion site clean and dry, and by removing the infusion set at the first signs of discomfort or redness;
    - unexplained hyperglycemia, usually resulting from a partial or complete interruption of insulin delivery that, if untreated, can lead to diabetic keto-acidosis; and
    - hypoglycemia, which can be reduced by monitoring blood glucose levels at least four times per day, weekly at 2:00–4:00 A.M., and before operating a motor vehicle.
- The insulin pump should be worn at all times. The patient should use an alternative insulin regimen if the pump is removed for >1–2 h.
- Successful insulin pump therapy requires thorough and ongoing education in technical components of the insulin pump and skills needed to adjust insulin for variations in daily activities.
- Insulin pump therapy in combination with a continuous glucose sensor can improve blood glucose control without increasing hypoglycemia.
- The future of diabetes treatment is promising thanks to advanced technologies that could lead to better information management systems, closed-loop insulin delivery systems, and further improvements in insulin pumps.

Diabetes Technology:
Insulin Infusion Pump Therapy and
Continuous Glucose Monitoring

T he search for optimal insulin regimens led to the development of technology such as insulin infusion pump therapy, which helps patients achieve diabetes self-management goals. Insulin infusion pumps deliver insulin continuously in a manner that approximates physiological insulin delivery and provides flexibility in day-to-day diabetes management. Along with continuous glucose monitoring (CGM), insulin pumps assist patients with diabetes to achieve near-normoglycemic control.

INSULIN INFUSION PUMP THERAPY

Continuous subcutaneous insulin infusion (CSII) includes a small pump, about the size of a beeper or cell phone, that contains a reservoir of short-acting (regular) or rapid-acting (insulin lispro, insulin aspart, insulin glulisine) insulin. Most patients use rapid-acting insulin in their insulin pumps. After filling the reservoir with a 2- to 3-day supply of the prescribed insulin, the reservoir is connected to an ~18- to 43-inch length of plastic tubing. At the end of the tubing is a 25- to 29-gauge needle or a soft Teflon cannula that the patient inserts into the subcutaneous tissue at a 30- to 45-degree or a 90-degree angle, depending on the type of infusion set used.

The exception to this is the Omnipod® pump, which is tubing free but has a built-in infusion set in the pod for insertion into the subcutaneous tissue. With the Omnipod®, the patient injects insulin into the pod before placement on the skin and insertion of the infusion needle. The pod has a self-adhesive backing that attaches to the skin. The pod, like the infusion sets, must be changed every 2–3 days.

The insulin pump delivers insulin in two ways. Basal insulin delivery is optimized to control hepatic glucose production and maintain stable glucose concentrations when the patient is fasting. In practice, most patients achieve glycemic goals using one to three different basal rates over a 24-h period. Depending on the model, insulin pumps can deliver basal rates from 0.025 to 35 units/h (in 0.025- to 5.0-unit increments).

Insulin is also delivered as a bolus, in anticipation of a meal, or to correct hyperglycemia. Depending on the pump manufacturer, the pump can deliver a 0.025- to 80-unit bolus (most deliver a maximum of 30–35 units) in 0.025- to 2-unit steps. Insulin pumps can be programmed to deliver a bolus over a longer period of time, often referred to as an extended or square-wave bolus. Patients, for example, can program their pump to deliver 4 units over a 3-h period to accommodate snacking (such as at a party) or for a high-fat meal. Patients also can program both a standard bolus and square-wave or extended bolus at the same time, also referred to as a dual-wave or combination bolus.

Insulin infusion pumps have therapeutic and safety features that facilitate achieving treatment goals in different situations. Depending on the pump manufacturer, patients can use their pumps to achieve several goals, including the following:

- Temporarily adjust the basal rate for periods of increased activity, illness, or stress without changing the usual basal rate program. The user can set the temporary basal rate in units or as a percentage of the usual basal rate.
- Suspend basal delivery if necessary. An "auto-off" is a safety feature that, if enabled, would suspend insulin delivery if no programming occurred within a specified period of time.
- Program several basal rate patterns (two to seven, depending on the pump model) so the patient can easily switch, for example, from a weekday to weekend pattern, premenstrual to postmenstrual pattern, high- to low-activity pattern, or day- to night-shift pattern.
- Review the amounts and times of previous boluses, which can be a valuable feature to avoid "stacking" of boluses and related hypoglycemia.
- Program boluses audibly or via a touch button or a shortcut button that bypasses the normal bolus screen.
- Program different insulin-to-carbohydrate ratios, different insulin sensitivity factors (ISFs), and different blood glucose targets by time of day.
- Use the pump's bolus calculator to determine insulin bolus requirements at mealtime and also to correct hyperglycemia. Most pumps calculate the amount of correction dose insulin depending on the time and amount of the previous insulin bolus to prevent stacking or overlapping doses of insulin. Use of bolus calculators eliminates the need for the patient to manually make these complex and time-consuming calculations.
- Set a missed meal bolus alert to remind patients to bolus for a meal. This is an important feature for patients who frequently miss insulin boluses.
- Set reminders on the pump to check blood glucose levels at specific times of day or if the blood glucose is above or below a specified level.

Some insulin pumps are watertight or water-resistant so that patients can wear their pumps while showering or engaging in some water sports, and this can be a practical consideration for some patients when choosing pump types. The size of the insulin reservoir varies in different pump types (with some holding up to 480 units), and the total daily insulin requirements of the patient also can be an important factor when choosing pumps. The American Diabetes Association publishes a consumer guide every year in their consumer magazine *Diabetes Forecast*. This guide provides current information on insulin pumps, blood glucose meters, and other diabetes management tools.

BENEFITS OF CSII

CSII leads to less dose-to-dose variability in insulin absorption than injections, and because of this, CSII is associated with less glycemic variability and risk for hypoglycemia. In practice, the basal infusion allows patients to skip or delay meals and maintain more stable glycemic control. The ability to give multiple meal insulin boluses can be a valuable convenience for more prolonged meals in restaurants or on social occasions. The ability to deliver meal boluses over an extended time can be a valuable feature for patients with gastroparesis, or when consuming high-fat meals that are associated with delayed gastric emptying and increased insulin requirements in the late postprandial period.

Basal infusion rates can be programmed to coincide with the diurnal variation of insulin sensitivity. Patients often need lower basal rates during the night (between ~11:00 P.M. and 3:00 A.M.) and higher basal rates between 3:00 or 4:00 A.M. and 9:00 A.M. to offset the effect of the dawn phenomenon and to prevent an increase in blood glucose levels in the morning. The basal rate can be adjusted temporarily during exercise, during the postexercise period when hypoglycemia is likely to occur, during illness, or before and during menses when insulin requirements tend to be higher.

Thus, insulin pump therapy optimizes the conditions for achieving good glycemic control while maintaining lifestyle flexibility. This therapeutic approach provides patients with the opportunity to fully participate in their self-care because they can make decisions about and adjustments to aspects of the regimen on a moment-to-moment basis as they encounter varying aspects of daily life.

Proper patient selection is critical to ensure the success of insulin pump therapy (see Table 7.1). Consider patients for insulin pump therapy

- to improve or stabilize glycemic control, especially if multiple daily insulin regimens have failed to solve self-management problems, such as wide glycemic excursions, nocturnal or frequent hypoglycemia, and effects of the dawn phenomenon;
- to increase lifestyle flexibility and deal with day-to-day variations in work or exercise schedule; or
- to meet increased self-management needs (i.e., to allow greater participation in self-care).

Patients who have erratic schedules, work different shifts, or travel frequently also can benefit from insulin pump therapy.

INITIAL DOSAGE CALCULATIONS FOR INSULIN PUMP THERAPY

Rapid-acting insulin has a quicker onset of action and a more pronounced peak of shorter duration than regular insulin. Rapid-acting insulin should be administered 5–15 min before ingestion of a meal, although to achieve optimal postprandial control, some higher glycemic index foods are best covered if the bolus is taken even earlier. Peak effectiveness of rapid-acting insulin occurs between 50 and 120 min after dosing as compared with 2–4 h for regular insulin. The more rapid onset and 1–2 h peak activity of the rapid-acting insulin can make correcting hyperglycemia simpler and quicker and lessens the likelihood that boluses taken close together will have overlapping action, leading to hypoglycemia. Most pumps calculate the amount of bolus insulin required depending on the time elapsed since the previous insulin bolus (called "insulin on board") to prevent stacking or overlapping doses of insulin.

Table 7.1 — Patient Selection Criteria for Insulin Pump Use

- Medical and metabolic indications, including
  - Suboptimal glycemic control using multiple daily injections
  - Wide blood glucose excursions
  - Different day versus night basal insulin requirements, including the dawn phenomenon
  - Frequent severe hypoglycemia
  - Nocturnal hypoglycemia
  - Pregnancy or planned conception
  - Gastroparesis
  - Variable daily schedule or lifestyle not well managed with multiple daily injections
- Patient demonstrates the technical and physical ability to
  - Perform blood glucose monitoring accurately and frequently (at least four times daily)
  - Perform the technical components of insulin pump use
  - Absence of serious disease or disability that would impair technical performance
- Patient demonstrates the intellectual ability to
  - Learn the technical and cognitive components of pump use (e.g., meal planning, the meaning of blood glucose levels, and adjusting insulin)
  - Determine the relationship between aspects of the regimen (e.g., food and insulin, activity and blood glucose levels)
- Patient demonstrates the motivation to
  - Perform frequent blood glucose monitoring to detect "unexplained" hyperglycemia, in particular to troubleshoot in the event of "unexplained" hyperglycemia that could be indicative of an insulin pump failure
  - Evaluate actions taken; engage in delivery problem
  - Keep follow-up appointments for therapy optimization
- Patient has the financial resources or a source of reimbursement for insulin pump, blood glucose monitoring supplies, and ongoing health care

BASAL INSULIN DOSAGE

Reduce pre-pump total daily dose (TDD) by 10–25% before calculating a starting basal rate. If the patient has a history of problematic hypoglycemia or hypoglycemia unawareness, it usually is prudent to be even more aggressive with dosage reductions.

For example, a patient with a glycated hemoglobin A_{1c} level of 7.2% takes a total daily dose of insulin (TDDI) of 55 units (reduce by 20%: 55 units × 0.20 = 11 units). Reduce the TDDI to 44 units (55 – 11) and divide by 2 (total basal dose should be 50% of TDDI: 44 units ÷ 2 = 22 units). Divide the total basal dose by 24 h (22 units ÷ 24 h = 0.92 units/h). The starting basal dose for this patient is 0.9 units/h.

An alternative method to calculate the total daily basal dose is to multiply the patient's weight in kilograms by 0.3–0.5. If the patient's weight is 176 lb (80 kg), the basal rate would be calculated as follows: (80 kg × 0.3 units/kg) ÷ 24 h = 1.0 unit/h.

Most patients with type 1 diabetes (T1D) require basal rates in the range of 0.4–2.0 units/h, with the average basal rate being 0.7–0.9 units/h. The average TDD for adults is 0.5–1.0 unit/kg body wt/day. Children usually require lower doses of insulin, whereas patients with type 2 diabetes (T2D) usually require more insulin.

Eliminate intermediate-acting insulin 12–24 h and long-acting insulin 24 h before initiating pump therapy. Instruct patients to take injections of short- or rapid-acting insulin, as needed, every 3–4 h to keep blood glucose levels reasonably controlled until pump therapy is begun.

Patients using insulin pump therapy have the advantage of programming different basal rates for varying diurnal insulin needs. Patients often need lower basal rates between bedtime and 3:00–4:00 A.M. and higher basal rates between 3:00 and 9:00 A.M. to deal with the dawn phenomenon. Patients may need an intermediate basal rate during the rest of the day. An adjustment of the basal rate by 10–20% is usually recommended. Using the previous example, if the patient's blood glucose profile revealed these varying diurnal insulin needs, the basal rate profile might be

- from 11:00 P.M. to 3:00 A.M., 0.9 units/h;
- from 3:00 A.M. to 7:00 A.M., 1.2 units/h; and
- from 7:00 A.M. to 11:00 P.M., 1.0 units/h.

Evaluate the basal rate using the 3:00 A.M. and fasting blood glucose levels and with basal check tests (i.e., omission of a meal with glucose checks performed every 2 h for a specific duration of time, usually 4–6 h). If these values are higher or lower than desired, adjust the basal rate accordingly, usually by increments of 0.05–0.2 units/h. If the 3:00 A.M. and fasting blood glucose levels are widely discrepant, the patient may need different basal rates during sleep and in the early morning (before waking) hours. Adjust the daytime basal rate based on basal check tests. For example, if the patient develops hypoglycemia when meals are skipped or delayed, the daytime basal rate is too high. In practice, changes in basal insulin infusion rates can take up to 2 h or longer to affect blood glucose concentrations, and this delay needs to be factored into the timing for adjustments of basal infusion rates.

BOLUS INSULIN DOSAGE

As a starting point, in optimizing prandial insulin dosing, bolus doses are calculated based on the number of grams of carbohydrate consumed. Preferably, the patient starting a pump has demonstrated competence in counting carbohydrates before the initiation of pump therapy. Ultimately, the goal is for the patient to be able to match the meal boluses to the intake of carbohydrate at each meal and snack with an individualized ratio of 1 unit of insulin per specific amount of carbohydrate. This is termed the "insulin-to-carbohydrate ratio."

During the first few days or weeks of pump therapy, it is useful to ask the patient to follow a prescribed meal plan based on the patient's usual dietary intake to establish the patient's insulin-to-carbohydrate ratio. It may be preferable to do this before initiating insulin pump therapy while the patient is using a multiple daily insulin injection regimen. Ask patients to keep detailed food records to help them master carbohydrate counting skills, demonstrate their ability and motivation to estimate carbohydrate intake, and determine their insulin-to-carbohydrate needs. Begin with a prescribed insulin dose for the meal plan and make adjustments until blood glucose levels are in the desired range. In some individuals, dietary fat can have a substantial effect on mealtime insulin requirements. Therefore, in practice, meals used to determine the patient's insulin-to-carbohydrate ratio ideally should be low fat.

As with all insulin regimens and adjustments, frequent blood glucose monitoring must be performed to determine the effectiveness of insulin dosages relative to accurate carbohydrate counting and bolus calculations and to the patient's usual activity level. Blood glucose monitoring should be done, initially, before each meal, within 1–2 h after the start of each meal, at bedtime, and at 2:00–4:00 A.M. until glycemic goals are achieved. Further adjustments will be required as the patient implements the insulin regimen under various situations.

The patient's ISF is used to adjust boluses to correct for premeal and between-meal hyperglycemia. To estimate the patient's ISF, divide 1,500 or 1,800 by the TDD. For example, a patient whose TDD is 46 units has an ISF of 40 mg/dL based on the following equation: $1,800 \div 46$ units = 39 mg/dL (round up to 40 mg/dL).

One unit of rapid-acting insulin is expected to decrease this patient's blood glucose by 40 mg/dL. Begin with a conservative estimate of the ISF. In general, patients who have diurnal changes in basal insulin requirements and different insulin-to-carbohydrate ratios for breakfast, lunch, and dinner will also require a different ISF for different time periods in the day. In practice, if basal insulin requirements during the dawn period are increased, the need for correction insulin dosages also will increase (i.e., lower ISF) during this time period. Conversely, if the basal insulin requirements during the early nocturnal period are lower, a corresponding need for correction insulin dosages also will decrease (i.e., higher ISF) during this time period.

When determining the amount of supplemental insulin, the patient should be advised to consider the time of the last bolus. If using regular insulin and the last bolus was taken <4 h ago, some percentage of activity from that bolus remains; therefore, reduce the supplemental insulin dose with that in mind (about 25% per hour). With rapid-acting insulin, peak pharmacodynamic activity is achieved in ~100 min, but the duration is still a concern if the patient is calculating a between-meal correction bolus. If the pump is programmed to calculate the bolus needs based on the patient's ISF, it will compute the insulin dose needed based on the time of the most recent bolus (i.e., insulin on board) to prevent stacking or overlapping insulin doses. If hypoglycemia from dose stacking is a problem, then the duration of action in the pump should be increased to 4 h or even longer. These adjustments will increase the assumed insulin on board used in the dosage calculations, leading to a reduction in the pump bolus recommendations.

Combining the insulin-to-carbohydrate ratio with the ISF, a patient with an insulin-to-carbohydrate ratio of 1 unit/10 g carbohydrate and an ISF of 1 unit/40 mg/dL would calculate a premeal bolus as follows (assuming the previous bolus was given beyond the programmed duration of insulin):

Blood glucose target is 110 mg/dL
ISF = 40
Blood glucose level = 179: 179 – 110 (target blood glucose) = 69;
    69 ÷ 40 (correction dose = 1.725 units)
Carbohydrate intake = 60 g: 60 ÷ 10
    (insulin-to-carbohydrate ratio is 1 unit/10 g) = 6 units of insulin
Calculated bolus is 6 + 1.7 = 7.7 units

INSULIN DOSAGE ADJUSTMENTS

DIET

Patients need to learn to adjust insulin boluses for variations in dietary intake so that blood glucose levels remain in the desired range. Usually 1 unit of insulin will cover 10–15 g carbohydrate. This can range from 0.5 to 2.0 units for every 10–15 g carbohydrate in patients with T1D. Patients, with the help of their clinician, will use food and glucose monitoring records to calculate the insulin-to-carbohydrate ratio, which may vary depending on the time of the meal (more insulin may be required at breakfast and less at lunch) or the type of food eaten. Precise estimates of the patient's insulin needs can be determined using detailed food, insulin, and blood glucose records. This is best calculated at the time the patient initiates intensive therapy when they are most interested in implementing their new therapy. Use detailed food records for a few days to a few weeks when initiating intensive therapy. Later in the course of managing insulin pump therapy, it can be useful to keep detailed food, insulin, and blood glucose records for a brief period, such as 3 days, to reevaluate the patient's insulin-to-carbohydrate ratio and to review carbohydrate counting. This evaluation may be necessary if the patient's weight or circumstances change or if the patient's blood glucose levels exceed target levels. Patients can be taught to count carbohydrate exchanges instead of counting carbohydrates by grams, and most pumps that have the capacity to calculate the patient's bolus can be programmed to match the insulin to starch exchanges or grams of carbohydrate.

A square-wave or extended bolus can be used when eating small amounts of food over an extended period of time, such as at a banquet or party, or when eating meals containing more slowly digested (lower glycemic index) carbohydrates such as pasta. The use of a square-wave or extended bolus may ensure better postprandial coverage in gastroparesis. Patients can program a normal bolus and square-wave or extended bolus at the same time (dual-wave or combination bolus). This approach might be useful for coverage of higher-fat foods, such as pizza, that are characterized by delayed gastric emptying and also late postprandial insulin resistance from free fatty acids. Research indicates that these meals are optimally covered by a combination bolus consisting of 10–50% initially with the remainder delivered over 2–3 h. To compensate for the insulin resistance from the free fatty acids, the total insulin dose will need to be more than that given for a meal with similar carbohydrate content but lower total fat. There are considerable interindividual differences in the amount of additional insulin that should be given for higher-fat meals; in practice, it is prudent to start with ~30% dose increase and then to adjust doses for future higher-fat meals as indicated based on a retrospective review of postprandial glucose profiles.

EXERCISE

CSII allows for greater flexibility in insulin dosing adjustments around exercise than multiple dose injection (MDI) therapy. The use of a temporary basal feature allows patients to minimize the need for carbohydrate intake around exercise, thereby allowing patients to more effectively use exercise as a strategy for weight control. Dosing adjustments need to be individualized based on the type, duration, and strenuousness of the activity. In general, decrease the premeal bolus by 25–50% for moderate levels of planned aerobic activity within 3 h of a meal. When exercising for sustained periods (>60 min), the patient may need to program a temporary basal rate reduction of 20–70%. At the conclusion of the exercise when muscle glucose uptake drops, the blood glucose may rebound (i.e., increase) because of ongoing accelerated hepatic glucose production resulting from the reduced basal insulin levels. The immediate reinstitution of basal insulin following exercise can be important in preventing this rebound hyperglycemia. Use of a temporary reduction in the basal rate after exercise also can be an effective strategy to avoid postexercise hypoglycemia that often occurs several hours after exercise.

Many pumps offer the ability to use a different set of 24-h basal rates that are most effective for exercise. For example, for planned exercise at specific times, the patient may choose to switch to his or her exercise-day program, which the patient presets with lower basal rates at specific times.

ILLNESS

Because hyperglycemia and ketosis from interruption of insulin delivery by pumps is often accompanied by nausea and abdominal discomfort, train patients who are beginning pump therapy that whenever they have a deterioration in metabolic control associated with physical symptoms, they must troubleshoot for insulin nondelivery (see the next section). For patients who take oral steroids, the basal rates of the pump can be adjusted to match the pharmacologic action of the steroids, thereby facilitating better glucose control than can be achieved using MDI. For example, if the patient is taking prednisone in the morning, basal rates from midmorning through late afternoon or early evening, as well as the meal and correction bolus doses for lunch and dinner programmed into the pump bolus calculator, would be increased.

RISKS OF CSII

SKIN INFECTION

Skin infections can occur at the infusion site and range from a small area of mild inflammation and tenderness to a large area of induration, inflammation, and soreness with purulent drainage. Antibiotics usually completely resolve the infections. Large abscesses may have to be surgically incised and drained.

To avoid infection, keep the infusion site clean and dry at all times. Soap and water usually are adequate to cleanse the skin before needle insertion. Patients who experience recurrent infusion site infections may need to use antibacterial cleansers. Known carriers of *Staphylococcus aureus* require antibacterial cleansers and meticulous care of the infusion site and may benefit from antibiotic treatment. Patients should be instructed to remove moist tape and to clean and dry the area around the needle insertion site. This procedure is especially important during the summer heat or during increased physical activity.

Insertion of sets in areas with visible scar tissue or areas where the underlying tissue feels hard or tough usually is associated with poor or unpredictable insulin absorption, especially following set insertion. Use of alternative nonscarred sites should be encouraged.

There are several types of infusion sets with various cannula and needle types, including straight or angled needles, needles attached to an adhesive disk, and Teflon cannulas with needle introducers. Pump infusion sets can be placed in the abdomen, hip, thigh, or upper arm. In practice, the abdomen is often the simplest and most comfortable. Because exercise can enhance insulin absorption, patients who are physically active may benefit from avoiding infusion catheter sites in exercising limbs. Teflon cannulas come in 6- to 17-mm lengths. Patients have a choice of cannula length and angle insertion, depending on their body type. Angled Teflon sets are less prone to kinking than perpendicular Teflon sets, especially in patients who are thin and have limited subcutaneous fat. In practice, the use of insertion devices with angled sets (such as the Sil-serterä or Inset 30ä) sometimes will lead to erratic insulin absorption, and angled sets are best inserted by hand. In contrast, use of insertion devices with perpendicular sets is not associated with this problem, and inserters are a valuable convenience that can enable patients to place infusion sets in areas such as the upper buttock that cannot be readily reached manually. Most cannula or infusion site problems, such as difficulty with needle insertion and skin breakdown, can be resolved by finding the type of cannula and tape or adhesive that best suits the individual patient. For patients who have frequent hyperglycemia resulting from the interruption of insulin delivery because of kinking of the Teflon infusion catheters, use of metal needle catheters can provide a practical solution.

Most infusion sets have self-adhesive tape; use of an additional adhesive dressing or surgical tape can help secure the needle or cannula and tubing in place. If patients are allergic to the self-adhesive infusion sets, find a tape or surgical dressing that does not cause a skin reaction or have the patient apply a protective solution or dressing (I.V. Prep Antiseptic Wipe, Tegaderm™, Skin-Tac™, Bard Protective Barrier Film®, Mastisol®, or Skin Bond™) before inserting the infusion set.

UNEXPLAINED HYPERGLYCEMIA AND KETOACIDOSIS

Because the insulin pump only uses rapid- or short-acting insulin, even a partial interruption of insulin delivery can rapidly result in hyperglycemia. Complete interruption of insulin delivery can result in ketosis or ketoacidosis within a few hours.

Patients new to insulin pump therapy must be taught to consider the possibility of interrupted insulin delivery any time high blood glucose levels persist for no apparent reason. In the absence of illness, if there has been no increase in dietary intake, no change in the insulin dose or timing, or no alteration in stress or activity levels, a disruption in insulin delivery should be suspected if hyperglycemia persists. The first indication of unexplained hyperglycemia often occurs with a routine blood glucose measurement, when the patient is surprised by an unusually high blood glucose value. If the blood glucose level has not decreased 2–4 h later after administering a correction bolus, the patient should troubleshoot to rule out interruption of insulin delivery. If urine ketones are also present or blood ketone (β-hydroxybutyrate) levels are increased, disruption of insulin delivery must be considered. Sometimes, the cause of unexplained hyperglycemia is insulin that has lost potency. This loss of potency should be suspected if no improvement in blood glucose levels are seen when the patient changes the reservoir and infusion set. If the patient administers an insulin bolus via a conventional syringe and the blood glucose level improves, the problem is with the insulin pump or the reservoir or pod, and not with the insulin.

There are many potential causes of unexplained hyperglycemia or ketoacidosis related to partial or complete failure of some component of the insulin infusion pump, syringe, or infusion set or pod (see Table 7.2). When a patient encounters a high blood glucose level (>250 mg/dL [>13.8 mmol/L]) that cannot be explained by an alteration in a component of the treatment plan, the patient should do a

---

Table 7.2—Unexplained Hyperglycemia: Factors to Consider

- Insulin pump
  - Basal rate programmed incorrectly
  - Battery depleted
  - Pump malfunction
  - Cartridge or syringe (reservoir) does not advance properly or pod is not functioning
  - Program or pump alarms
  - Program functions cannot be set
- Cartridge or syringe (reservoir)
  - Improper placement in the pump
  - Empty cartridge or syringe (insulin depleted)
  - Leakage of insulin
  - Cartridge or syringe not positioned to advance and infuse
  - Did not prime reservoir or infusion set correctly
- Infusion set and needle or cannula
  - Insulin leakage
  - Dislodged needle, cannula, or pod
  - Bent or kinked cannula or incorrect cannula or pod insertion
  - Insulin not administered to account for dead space after introducer needle is removed when infusion cannula is inserted
  - Air in infusion set tubing
  - Blood in infusion set tubing
  - Occlusion at the site
  - Infusion set in place >48–72 h
  - Tear in the tubing
  - Occlusion of the insulin in the infusion set
  - Loose cartridge or syringe and infusion set connection
- Infusion site
  - Redness, irritation, inflammation, induration
  - Discomfort
  - Placement in an area of hypertrophy or scar tissue
  - Placement in an area of friction or near the belt line
- Insulin
  - Has clumped particles or crystallized appearance
  - Is beyond expiration date
  - Was exposed to extreme temperatures
  - Vial has been used for >1 month or is nearly empty
  - Prior bolus inadequate for carbohydrate consumed

systematic investigation of the pump, cartridge or syringe, infusion set or pod, infusion site, and insulin to identify the cause. If the patient detects a problem with the site, the infusion set tubing, or the connection between the syringe and the infusion set, immediately change the cannula or pod and site. If a problem with the pump is identified, reprogram the pump or contact the pump manufacturer to troubleshoot the problem or replace the pump if it is within the warranty period.

If no obvious cause is found, assume that there is an infusion problem, most likely caused by kinking of the infusion set or scarring of the infusion site, and replace the pump reservoir and infusion set or pod and change the site. If the pump is inoperable or malfunctioning, patients should use a multicomponent injection regimen until the pump can be replaced (see Chapter 6). All patients should know how to use an alternative insulin regimen with conventional insulin syringes in case a problem with the pump or some component of the infusion system occurs. Instruct patients to always carry extra insulin, pump supplies (batteries, infusion sets, and pump cartridges, syringes, or pods), and conventional syringes or an insulin pen delivery device. In case of hospitalization, it is best to be prepared to carry in these supplies, in case the hospital policy will permit self-management to continue, under the conditions of the hospitalization.

When the patient detects unexplained hyperglycemia and corrects the problem, then the hyperglycemia and ketonuria must be treated. The patient should monitor blood glucose and urine or blood ketone levels every 1–3 h. Advise the patient to take insulin boluses in amounts determined by the patient's insulin sensitivity and daily insulin requirements until urine ketones have cleared (or blood ketone levels are <0.6 mmol/L) and blood glucose levels have returned to the desired range. The patient who develops nausea and vomiting and is unable to maintain fluid intake should go to an emergency room for treatment.

HYPOGLYCEMIA

A lower incidence of hypoglycemia has been observed with insulin pump therapy as compared with multiple daily injections. Strategies to avoid hypoglycemia and methods of teaching hypoglycemia awareness are essentially the same for any intensive diabetes management approach, regardless of the mode of insulin delivery. Patients should have a source of rapidly absorbed carbohydrate, such as juice, regular soda, or glucose tablets, with them at all times, including at work, in the car, at the gym, and at the bedside. Encourage patients to check their blood glucose levels before operating machinery or a motor vehicle. All patients using a pump should have glucagon and a close family member or friend instructed on its use. To avoid accidentally infusing insulin, advise patients to disconnect the infusion set tubing before removing a used cartridge or reservoir (syringe) or replacing an infusion set. The patient should not use the prime, load, or fill tubing feature while an infusion set is connected to the body. Another major issue that can contribute to risk for hypoglycemia in pump users is incorrectly set basal rates, in particular, inadvertent increases in basal rates to cover food-related elevations in the blood glucose. For example, patients noticing consistent elevations in their blood glucoses in the late evening period because of snacking commonly will increase the basal rates rather than take additional bolus insulin; however, on occasions when evening eating is delayed or food intake is less, hypoglycemia will occur.

Avoiding severe hypoglycemia begins with selecting patients who are good candidates for intensive therapy (see Table 7.3). Patients must be prepared to check blood glucose levels at least four times a day to monitor pump operation

Table 7.3—Education for Insulin Pump Therapy

Phase 1: Choosing insulin pump therapy (one or two outpatient visits)

- Components of insulin pump therapy
- Advantages and disadvantages of insulin pump therapy
- Financial requirements
- Goals of therapy
- Carbohydrate counting
- Suitability for insulin pump use (this can include a several-month trial of frequent blood glucose monitoring, trial of multiple daily insulin injections, carbohydrate counting, and use of insulin sensitivity or correction factor)

Phase 2: Initiating insulin pump therapy

- Several sessions with health-care team over several months, a 2- to 4-h technical training session with pump trainer, and a visit with health-care provider
- Technical components of the insulin pump (see Table 7.4)
- Blood glucose–monitoring technique and accuracy confirmed
- Carbohydrate counting review and fine-tuning skills to establish insulin-to-carbohydrate ratio
- Symptoms, prevention, and treatment of hypoglycemia
- Optional trial of wearing the insulin pump using normal saline
- Determination of initial starting basal rate

Phase 3: Postinitiation of insulin pump therapy

- Daily phone contact for 7–10 days and biweekly follow-up visits for first 2–4 weeks; maintain close contact for 2–6 months; have patient keep food, blood glucose, and insulin records
- Focus on mastering blood glucose monitoring, calculating meal boluses based on carbohydrate counting, calculating correction bolus doses based on glucose monitoring, and insulin pump operation
- Fine-tune insulin dosages to achieve blood glucose goals
- Identify relationships between blood glucose readings and food intake, activity, and insulin
- Adjust aspects of the regimen to meet lifestyle needs based on patient input
- Assist patient to integrate the treatment plan into daily life

Ongoing follow-up

- Continuing visits every 1–3 months of 30–60 min using all team members as needed
- Interpreting blood glucose readings
- Adjusting insulin for variations in dietary intake and activity
- Using the pump and advanced pump options to deal with varying situations
- Dealing with pump-related problems
- Adapting treatment recommendations to changes in lifestyle
- Anticipating situations that could cause alterations in glycemic control
- Identifying obstacles to implementing treatment recommendations and developing strategies to overcome obstacles
- Setting and evaluating treatment and blood glucose goals

and to make and evaluate decisions regarding insulin doses. Patients often take insulin without checking their blood glucose levels, a practice that increases the risk of hypoglycemia. This should be discouraged. Patients should be encouraged to carry their blood glucose testing equipment with them at all times. Physical capabilities to program the pump and monitor its operation are necessary; patients must be able to understand the relationships between components of the treatment plan and their effects on blood glucose levels. Anticipating insulin needs for varying activities increases the likelihood that patients will make the appropriate adjustments in insulin so that blood glucose levels remain in the desired range.

WEARING THE PUMP

During patient training, it needs to be reinforced that the pump must be worn at all times. Removing the pump for >1–2 h without insulin compensation puts the patient at risk for developing hyperglycemia and ketosis. Patients frequently are concerned about initiating insulin pump therapy because they believe that it will interfere with activities they enjoy. The pump can be worn during most activities, with the exception of contact sports. Because of the effect of heat on insulin stability, pumps should not be submerged in hot tubs and should not be exposed to high temperatures during long periods of time outdoors during the summer. If the pump is not watertight, it must be removed for showering or placed in a plastic sheath. If engaging in certain water sports, the patient can remove the pump or place the pump in a waterproof holder. Some pumps are watertight for unlimited surface activity and are considered watertight only up to certain water depths and for specified periods of time.

Most patients are concerned about what to do with the insulin pump during sexual activity, but they may not feel comfortable asking about it. If the patient does not bring up the topic, initiate a discussion about sexual activity and pump use. Most couples find that wearing the insulin pump during sexual activity does not interfere with sexual intimacy. If the pump is disconnected during sexual activity, caution the patient to resume insulin pump delivery within an hour or so. After sexual activity, check the tape and infusion set or pod to ensure that the system is intact and secure. Following are alternatives for patients who do not wish to wear their pumps for certain periods of time, including days at the beach, vacations, or an evening out:

- If using an infusion set with a disconnect feature, disconnect the pump for up to 1–2 h depending on the level of activity (leave the needle or cannula in place).
- Take injections of rapid- or short-acting insulin before meals and wear the pump at night to provide basal insulin needs; or take an injection of basal insulin to cover most basal insulin requirements during the day when the pump is removed, and use the pump for boluses and to provide additional basal coverage for the dawn period.

Remind patients that there are some limitations on the timing of insulin and meals while off the pump. More blood glucose monitoring should be performed while using an alternative insulin regimen.

When traveling by air, patients usually do not have problems with airport security while wearing an insulin pump. Patients may request a letter from their health-care provider that documents their need for an insulin pump, pump supplies, and blood glucose monitoring equipment. Because patients cannot carry liquids, such as juice or soda, through airport security, they should carry glucose tablets and then purchase juice or soda after getting through security, if necessary. Patients who have very tightly controlled blood glucose levels should be aware that changes in altitude have been shown to cause unintended insulin delivery from their pumps. During takeoff, when air pressure decreases, pumps can deliver additional insulin, whereas during descent the converse can occur.

PATIENT EDUCATION FOR CSII

Appropriate education for insulin pump therapy takes place in three phases (see Table 7.3). The first phase occurs before initiating pump therapy. During this period, discuss the advantages and disadvantages of pump therapy, the patient's personal treatment goals, and the patient's resources to successfully manage insulin pump therapy. As indicated, initiate strategies to establish the patient's suitability for insulin pump use, such as a trial of performing and recording four blood glucose tests per day, using a multiple daily insulin regimen with carbohydrate counting, or adding insulin algorithms to an existing insulin regimen before establishing the patient's ISF. With the health-care provider's assistance, the patient should choose the pump brand and model and verify insurance coverage and requirements. For example, before approving an insulin pump, some insurance companies require several weeks or months of blood glucose records and an A1C level.

After the decision to initiate insulin pump therapy is made, the second phase of education begins. During this period, verify blood glucose–monitoring and nutrition knowledge and self-management skills. This education can be accomplished through a series of outpatient visits with certified diabetes educators (nurses and nutritionists). The patient can be given the opportunity to wear the pump for several days, using normal saline to master the technical skills associated with pump therapy and to increase his or her comfort with the idea of wearing a pump. In general, most pump initiations are done on an outpatient basis. If pump initiation and education are offered on an outpatient basis, the patient will need to perform frequent blood glucose monitoring and maintain close contact with the health-care team. This contact usually consists of daily phone calls or faxing or e-mailing blood glucose results, carbohydrate counting, and bolus dose records. Focus on teaching the basic components of insulin pump therapy, including the technical components of the pump (see Table 7.4), the pump's insulin delivery system, carbohydrate counting, monitoring blood glucose, and preventing and treating hypoglycemia and hyperglycemia.

The third phase begins after insulin doses are determined and the patient demonstrates technical competence using the pump. This phase is an intensive period of follow-up lasting 2–6 months, during which time the patient masters the skills learned in the second phase and integrates those skills into the usual activities of

Table 7.4 – Technical Components of Insulin Pump Therapy

- Pump operation
  - Placement of the battery or batteries
  - Programming the meal bolus and extended or square-wave bolus
  - Programming basal rates
  - Preparation and placement of insulin cartridge or syringe and infusion set or pod (priming infusion set)
  - Infusion site selection, rotation, and care
  - Meaning of alarms and how to respond
  - Programming additional basal rates and basal rate programs as needed and temporary basal rate changes
  - Programming additional pump options (e.g., beep or vibrate, bolus calculator, quick bolus options, setting alarms, and history features)
  - Troubleshooting
- Self-monitoring of blood glucose
  - Determining proper technique
  - Confirming accuracy of results
  - Interpreting blood glucose readings
  - Setting blood glucose goals
  - Using linked meter to help calculate required insulin dosages based on personal settings
- Carbohydrate counting and learning relationship between insulin and food
- Using insulin sensitivity or correction factor
- Learning about hypoglycemia and hyperglycemia: symptoms, causes, prevention, and treatment
- Learning about unexplained hyperglycemia: causes, prevention, identification, and treatment
- Managing sick days
- Dealing with exercise
- Determining options for special occasions
- Deciding on an insulin regimen when insulin pump use is not desired or pump malfunctions
- Determining decision-making strategies for dealing with lifestyle changes

daily life. Visits with a member of the health-care team may take place every 2–3 weeks in addition to weekly phone contact. The patient should keep blood glucose and food records to facilitate learning to quantify food and plan meals and to identify relationships among blood glucose levels, insulin dose and timing, dietary intake, and activity. These records also enable the health-care team to modify insulin doses and determine whether the patient understands all of the components of the treatment plan. Some issues to consider when educating the patient with erratic glucose control are listed in Table 7.5.

REAL-TIME CONTINUOUS GLUCOSE MONITORING

In the past decade real-time continuous glucose monitoring (RT-CGM) has become a routine part of intensive management in adults and also children with T1D. Several trials have demonstrated that, in contrast to intervention studies

Table 7.5—Practical Issues to Consider in the Pump Patient with Erratic Glucose Control

Several pump-specific issues can cause erratic glucose control in the pump user. In the course of follow up visits the clinician should routinely:

1. Examine pump infusion sites. Scarring and lipohypertrophy of infusion sites are not uncommon causes for unpredictable glucoses, especially in long-term pump users.
2. Ask whether the patient has had catheter kinking or dislodgement. Plastic catheters that are perpendicular to the skin surface are more prone to kink or become dislodged, especially with activity and perspiration. Solutions include use of antiperspirants or changing to metal needle infusion sets, plastic sets with a shorter cannula, or other types of plastic infusion sets that are less prone to kinking. These include sets that insert obliquely such as the Silouette™ and Comfort™. Note of caution: Practical experience indicates that use of insertion devices with oblique catheters (such as the Silserter™ or Inset 30™ [which has an integrated inserter]) often are associated with erratic glucose control, presumably because of tissue trauma; patients should be encouraged to insert these oblique catheters manually. Patients using Teflon catheters who have inexplicable glucose fluctuations should be offered a trial with a metal needle catheter.
3. Ask whether the patient changes the pump reservoir and infusion system on a regular basis. This can be confirmed with the pump download. In reviewing the pump and glucose data, check for the tendency for elevated and erratic glucose in the period preceding infusion set changes. Insulin instability in the pump infusion system can manifest as higher glucoses if the reservoir and catheter is kept in place for too long or even precipitation in the infusion system. A study comparing insulin stability in pumps placed in an incubator at a temperature to 32–36°C to simulate the clinical environment showed an increased rate of catheter occlusions from day 3 to day 5 with more occlusions for glulisine compared with lispro and aspart insulin. Practical experience indicates that some patients with erratic glucose levels who are prescribed a change in insulin type or more frequent catheter and infusion system changes will demonstrate improved glycemic control. Routines need to be individualized, however, and some patients with stable and good glycemic control can safely use reservoirs and catheters for longer than mandated by the label.

Review of pump downloads can help identify the possible causes for erratic glucoses. In reviewing the data, the clinician should

- check priming history of the pump to assess how frequently the infusion system is being changed, and examine whether delayed set changes are associated with increased glucose levels;
- check percentage of basal to bolus insulin—a high percentage of basal insulin in the patient with frequent hyperglycemia may point to possibility that bolus doses are being missed, whereas a high percentage of basal insulin in the patient with frequent hypoglycemia may indicate that basal rates are too high and are contributing to the hypoglycemia; and
- check bolus history to detect possible missed meal boluses and also determine whether boluses are being delivered to correct hyperglycemia.

(such as the Diabetes Control and Complications Trial) in which patients used intermittent capillary glucose monitoring to guide diabetes self-management, use of RT-CGM by patients with T1D can lead to a reduction in A1C *without* an associated increase in hypoglycemia. Current RT-CGM devices approved for long-term clinical use have transcutaneous sensors that measure the glucose concentration every few minutes. These devices generally are less accurate than current fingerstick capillary blood glucose meters; however, this limitation is offset by the additional information about the rate and direction of changes in the glucose level and glucose patterns as well as alarms that are triggered by both hyper- and hypoglycemia. The data from the glucose sensor is displayed on a receiver unit or smartphone (Dexcom G4 and G5ä) or insulin pump (Animas, Medtronic, and Tandem pumps).

To use RT-CGM technology safely and effectively, patients need to have advanced diabetes self-management skills and must understand several key concepts (including physiologic lag). Currently available CGM devices measure glucose in the interstitial fluid in the subcutaneous tissue, whereas glucose meters measure capillary blood glucose obtained by fingerstick. When the glucose concentration is changing, there is a physiologic lag in the equilibration of glucose between these two compartments. This lag has important implications for the accuracy of continuous glucose sensors and the use of RT-CGM in diabetes self-management. RT-CGM does not eliminate the need for fingerstick capillary blood glucose measurements. These measurements are required to calibrate the sensor and confirm glucose readings before an insulin bolus. The alarms for hypo- and hyperglycemia are an important feature of RT-CGM devices. To ensure that the patient derives maximum benefit from use of the alarms, the alarm thresholds must be individualized. If alarm thresholds are set at the "ideal" level (e.g., low = 90 mg/dL, high = 180 mg/dL), the patient will be warned of most low and high glucose values; however, they also will experience frequent false alarms with increased risk for "alarm burnout" and a related tendency to ignore the alarms. Conversely, if alarm thresholds are set more widely (e.g., low = 60 mg/dL, high = 240 mg/dL), the patient will experience few false alarms and less risk for "alarm burnout," but they will not be warned about all low and high glucose values. During clinic follow-up visits, review alarms to determine whether the patient is getting the necessary alarms when the glucose is low, especially during the nocturnal period when vulnerability to hypoglycemia is the greatest. If the patient is having frequent, intermittent fasting hyperglycemia but the high alarm is not going off, the high alarm threshold may need to be reduced.

The insights gained from CGM about postprandial glucose patterns can help optimize diabetes management. For example, higher glycemic index carbohydrate breakfast foods (such as cold cereal) lead to a rapid postprandial spike, and uncovering this pattern will focus attention on the need for early premeal bolusing or even prompt a change to alternative lower glycemic index breakfast foods. Some patients will overreact to postprandial glucose spikes identified by the CGM by taking excessive additional insulin boluses, and the resultant dose stacking can lead to hypoglycemia. During the initial training when patients start on RT-CGM, they should be cautioned about the risks from overbolusing and about the need to consider residual insulin on board from the premeal bolus before taking additional insulin.

Although sensor-augmented insulin pumps (i.e., insulin pumps that have integrated RT-CGM devices) have been available for a decade, thus far, there have not been any large randomized controlled trials comparing sensor-augmented pump therapy directly to MDI with RT-CGM. Sensor-augmented insulin pump technology has been further enhanced with a low-glucose-suspend feature, in which the pump can be programmed to discontinue insulin delivery when the sensor glucose reaches a certain threshold. In one study in adults with documented nocturnal hypoglycemia, patients randomly assigned to a sensor-augmented pump with the low-glucose-suspend feature had an overall reduction in nocturnal hypoglycemia. Ongoing research with the use of prediction algorithms that trigger the reduction of the pump basal rates in advance of hypoglycemia hold further promise in minimizing the risk for hypoglycemia associated with intensive diabetes management.

CONCLUSION

Insulin pump therapy provides many advantages for patients with diabetes who are seeking improved glycemic control with less risk for hypoglycemia as well as increased lifestyle flexibility. More physiologic insulin delivery, less variability in insulin absorption, and several technical features that enable patients to modify insulin delivery according to their specific lifestyle requirements make insulin pump therapy an ideal treatment option for individuals seeking greater flexibility and more control over their diabetes self-management. Careful dosing and adjustment of basal and bolus insulin delivery, comprehensive patient education, and ongoing follow-up are essential for successful insulin pump therapy. RT-CGM can help patients further to reduce glycemic variability and risk for hypoglycemia. The future is promising as improved technologies are applied to diabetes management.

BIBLIOGRAPHY

Attia N, Jones TW, Holcombe J, Tamborlane WV. Comparison of human regular and lispro insulins after interruption of continuous subcutaneous insulin infusion and in the treatment of acutely decompensated IDDM. *Diabetes Care* 1998;21:817–821

Bailey T, Ellis S, Garg S, Kaplan R, Jovanovic L, Schwartz S, Zisser H. Improvement in glycemic excursions with a transcutaneous real-time continuous glucose sensor. *Diabetes Care* 2006;29:44–50

Bell KJ, Smart CE, Steil GM, Brand-Miller JC, King B, Wolpert HA. Impact of fat, protein and glycemic index on postprandial glucose control in type 1 diabetes: implications for intensive diabetes management in the continuous glucose monitoring era. *Diabetes Care* 2015;38:1008–1015

Bergenstal RM, Klonoff DC, Garg SK, et al. Threshold-based insulin-pump interruption for reduction of hypoglycemia. *N Engl J Med* 2013;369:224–232

Bergenstal RM, Tamborlane WV, Ahmann A, Buse JB, Dailey G, Davis SN, et al. Effectiveness of sensor-augmented insulin-pump therapy in type 1 diabetes. *N Engl J Med* 2010;363:311–320

Bode BW, Garg S, Hirsch IB, Hu P, Kolaczynski JW, Lane WS, Santiago OM, Sussman A. Continuous subcutaneous insulin infusion (CSII) of insulin aspart versus multiple daily injection of insulin aspart/insulin glargine in type 1 diabetic patients previously treated with CSII. *Diabetes Care* 2005;28:533–538

Bode BW, Tamborlane WV, Davidson PC. Insulin pump therapy in the 21st century: strategies for successful use in adults, adolescents, and children with diabetes (Review). *Postgrad Med* 2002;111:69–77

Corriveau EA, Durso PJ, Kaufman ED, Skipper BJ, Laskaratos LA, Heintzman KB. Effect of Carelink, an internet-based insulin pump monitoring system, on glycemic control in rural and urban children with type 1 diabetes mellitus. *Pediatr Diabetes* 2008;9:360–366

Dassau E, Cameron F, Lee H, Bequette BW, Zisser H, Jovanovic L, Chase HP, Wilson DM, Buckingham BA, Doyle FJ III. Real-time hypoglycemia prediction suite using continuous glucose monitoring. A safety net for the artificial pancreas. *Diabetes Care* 2010;33:1249–1254

Dassau E, Jovanovic L, Doyle FJ 3rd, Zisser HC. Enhanced 911/global position system wizard: a telemedicine application for the prevention of severe hypoglycemia—monitor, alert, and locate. *J Diabetes Sci Tech* 2009;3:1501–1506

Diabetes Control and Complications Trial (DCCT) Research Group. Implementation of treatment protocols in the Diabetes Control and Complications Trial. *Diabetes Care* 1995;18:361–376

Diabetes Control and Complications Trial (DCCT) Research Group. Hypoglycemia in the Diabetes Control and Complications Trial. *Diabetes* 1997;46:271–286

Golden SH, et al. AHRQ comparative effectiveness reviews. In *Methods for Insulin Delivery and Glucose Monitoring: Comparative Effectiveness*. Agency for Healthcare Research and Quality (US), Rockville, MD, 2012

Grunberger G, et al. Consensus statement by the American Association of Clinical Endocrinologists/American College of Endocrinology Insulin Pump Management Task Force. *Endocr Pract* 2014;20:463–489

Hirsch IB. Algorithms for care in adults using continuous glucose monitoring. *J Diabetes Sci Technol* 2007;1:126–129

Hirsch IB, Abelseth J, Bode BW, Fischer JS, Kaufman FR, Mastrototaro J, Parkin CG, Wolpert HA, Buckingham BA. Sensor-augmented insulin pump therapy: results of the first randomized treat-to-target study. *Diabetes Technol Ther* 2008;10:377–383

Hirsch IB, Armstrong D, Bergenstal RM, Buckingham B, Childs BP, Clarke WL, Peters A, Wolpert H. Clinical application of emerging sensor technologies in diabetes management: consensus guidelines for continuous glucose monitoring (CGM). *Diabetes Technol Therapeut* 2008;10:232–246

Juvenile Diabetes Research Foundation Continuous Glucose Monitoring Study Group. Continuous glucose monitoring and intensive treatment of type 1 diabetes. *N Engl J Med* 2008;359:1464–1476

Juvenile Diabetes Research Foundation Continuous Glucose Monitoring Study Group. The effect of continuous glucose monitoring in well-controlled type 1 diabetes. *Diabetes Care* 2009;32:1378–1383

Keen H, Pickup J. Continuous subcutaneous insulin infusion at 25 years. *Diabetes Care* 2002;25:593–598

King BR, Goss PW, Paterson MA, Crock PA, Anderson DG. Changes in altitude cause unintended insulin delivery from insulin pumps: mechanisms and implications. *Diabetes Care* 2011;34:1932–1933

Kerr D, Morton J, Whately-Smith C, Everett J, Begley JP. Laboratory-based non-clinical comparison of occlusion rates using three rapid-acting insulin analogs in continuous subcutaneous insulin infusion catheters using low flow rates. *J Diabetes Sci Technol* 2008;2:450–455

Kovatchev B, Cobelli C, Renard E, Anderson S, Breton M, Patek S, Clarke W, Bruttomesso D, Maran A, Costa S, Avogaro A, Dalla Mann C, Facchinetti A, Magni L, DeNicolao G, Place J, Farret A. Multinational study of subcutaneous model-predictive closed-loop control in type 1 diabetes mellitus: Summary of the results. *J Diabetes Sci Tech* 2010;4:1374–1381

Lenhard MJ, Reeves GD. Continuous subcutaneous insulin infusion: a comprehensive review of insulin pump therapy. *Arch Intern Med* 2001;161:2293–2300

Phillip M, Battelino T, Rodriguez H, Danne T, Kaufman F. Use of insulin pump therapy in the pediatric age group: consensus statement from the European Society for Paediatric Endocrinology, the Lawson Wilkins Pediatric Endocrine Society, and the International Society for Pediatric and Adolescent Diabetes, endorsed by the American Diabetes Association and the European Association for the Study of Diabetes. *Diabetes Care* 2007;30:1653–1662

Pickup J, Keen H. Continuous subcutaneous insulin infusion at 25 years: evidence base for the expanding use of insulin pump therapy in type 1 diabetes (Review). *Diabetes Care* 2002;25:593–598

Pickup J, Sutton A. Severe hypoglycaemia and glycaemic control in type 1 diabetes: meta-analysis of multiple daily insulin injections compared with continuous subcutaneous insulin infusion. *Diabet Med* 2008;25:765–774

Shetty G, Wolpert H. Insulin pump use in adults with type 1 diabetes—practical issues. *Diabetes Technol Therapeut* 2010;12(Suppl. 1):S11–S16

Walsh J, Roberts R. *Pumping Insulin*. 4th ed. San Diego, CA, Torrey Pines Press, 2007

Wang Y, Dassau E, Zisser H, Jovanovic L, Doyle F III. Automatic bolus and adaptive basal algorithm for the artificial pancreatic β-cell. *Diabetes Technol Ther* 2010;12:879–887

Wolpert HA, Faradji RN, Bonner-Weir S, Lipes MA. Metabolic decompensation in pump users due to lispro insulin precipitation. *BMJ* 2002;324:1253

Wolpert H. The nuts and bolts of achieving end points with real-time continuous glucose monitoring. *Diabetes Care* 2008;31(Suppl. 2):S146–S149

Wolpert H, Atakov-Castillo A, Smith S, Steil G. Dietary fat acutely increases glucose concentrations and insulin requirements in patients with type 1 diabetes: implications for carbohydrate-based bolus dose calculation and intensive diabetes management. *Diabetes Care* 2003;36:810–816

Monitoring

DOI: 10.2337/9781580406321.08

Highlights
Monitoring

- Regular monitoring is an essential component of any diabetes regimen. During intensive diabetes management, monitoring is even more important and must be done more frequently than during conventional treatment.

- Monitoring during intensive diabetes management includes self-monitoring of blood glucose (SMBG) as well as urine and blood ketone monitoring.

- Monitoring of blood glucose during symptoms of hypoglycemia is strongly recommended, as is monitoring before driving an automobile.

- Monitoring of metabolic control by the health-care team at each visit should include
  - glycated hemoglobin A_{1c}—estimated average glucose;
  - review of blood glucose data; and
  - assessment of growth, weight, and blood pressure.

- Converting A1C measurements into an estimated average glucose value helps "translate" the A1C into a number patients can understand, and makes treatment goals more tangible.

- Monitoring the development and progression of long-term complications of diabetes should be performed at least as often as proposed by the American Diabetes Association in its Standards of Medical Care (see the section Monitoring for Long-Term Complications).

Monitoring

R egular monitoring is an essential component of any diabetes management regimen. In intensive diabetes management, monitoring is even more important and must be done more frequently than in conventional treatment regimens. This is true for both the medical monitoring performed by the health-care team and the day-to-day monitoring required by the patient. Patient monitoring includes self-monitoring of blood glucose (SMBG) and ketone monitoring. Monitoring by health-care providers includes regular determination of glycated hemoglobin A_{1c}, careful assessment of growth and development (in both children and adolescents) and weight (in adults), careful review of hypoglycemia episodes and related complications, review of ketone monitoring and sick-day management, and monitoring for the presence of long-term diabetes complications.

MONITORING BY THE PATIENT

All patients using an intensive diabetes management program need to perform monitoring on a daily basis at home, work, school, or wherever they may be.

BLOOD GLUCOSE

When implementing an intensive diabetes management regimen, patients often will perform SMBG four to six times a day. An inability or unwillingness to perform SMBG should be considered a contraindication to implementing intensive diabetes therapy. A reasonable expectation should be for at least three to four SMBG determinations a day. An intensive diabetes management regimen rarely can be optimally successful without monitoring blood glucose at least four times a day, and should not be recommended if the patient performs fewer than three blood glucose determinations a day.

The four essential SMBG determinations for successful implementation of an intensive diabetes management regimen must be performed before each meal and before bedtime. Premeal measurements are needed to determine the dose of insulin or meal or activity alterations required to achieve the target glucose level over the next few hours. These measurements also are used to determine patterns of glycemia over time that will guide adjustment of the regimen. It is best to observe these patterns over periods of at least 3–5 days before making an overall change in the regimen. The bedtime blood glucose measurement is essential to assess the adequacy of the dinnertime dose of insulin and is also a key safety component in preventing nocturnal hypoglycemia. The morning value is used to assess the adequacy of overnight glycemic control.

Recent reports stress the importance of postprandial glycemia to achieve and maintain target A1C values and to prevent micro- and macrovascular disease complications. Two- to three-hour postprandial glucose determinations are essential to determine optimal meal insulin doses. After the appropriate meal insulin doses have been determined, postprandial monitoring for each meal remains important and should be performed at least once a week to verify the correct bolus or meal insulin doses.

In addition to these four blood glucose determinations, monitoring should include a periodic blood glucose measurement between 2:00 and 4:00 A.M. to detect unrecognized nocturnal hypoglycemia. This monitoring is especially important following more active days and for patients in whom the target blood glucose range is near the nondiabetic range, or for patients in whom nocturnal or severe hypoglycemia or hypoglycemia unawareness has been a problem. Nocturnal monitoring may need to be performed more often than once a week during periods when the basal insulin dose is being adjusted.

Monitoring blood glucose when symptoms of hypoglycemia occur is strongly recommended. Because hypoglycemia can occur with few or no early warning symptoms (hypoglycemia unawareness), and because autonomic (adrenergic) symptoms can occur in the absence of hypoglycemia, patient should confirm biochemical hypoglycemia and measure their blood glucose level when symptoms occur.

Because some patients' driving ability may be impaired at blood glucose levels higher than those that usually trigger easily recognizable hypoglycemia symptoms (especially in patients with hypoglycemia unawareness and those using intensive diabetes therapy), it is strongly recommended that blood glucose be monitored before driving.

KETONE MONITORING

Monitoring for the presence of ketones is an essential component of diabetes care. In certain situations ketone monitoring is necessary for the safe implementation of diabetes therapy, regardless of the type of therapy used (see Table 8.1).

Ketone monitoring can be done using strips that measure urine ketones (acetoacetate and acetone) or with a meter that measures blood β-hydroxybutyrate concentration. This device is similar to other SMBG meters and also can measure blood glucose levels using a different strip in the same meter. The advantages of urine-monitoring strips include ease of sample collection under most circumstances and low cost. Measurement of blood ketones offers the special advantage in young children who may not cooperate during urine ketone testing, especially during illness. Additionally, during a gastrointestinal illness, modest dehydration may result in concentrated urine, causing the urine ketone determination to indicate severe ketonuria, even though the blood ketone value is not markedly elevated. Under these circumstances, measurement of blood ketone levels may prevent a trip to the emergency room. Blood ketone determination is significantly more expensive than urine ketone determination, but in some circumstances, it may be cost-effective.

Table 8.1—Patient Monitoring During Intensive Diabetes Management

- Self-monitoring of blood glucose
  - Before each meal
  - At bedtime
  - Between 2:00 and 4:00 A.M. at least weekly
  - When symptoms of hypoglycemia occur
  - Before driving
- Ketone monitoring
  - During any illness
  - During unexpected or persistent hyperglycemia
  - Daily during pregnancy
  - For patients on sodium-glucose linked transporter (SGLT) inhibitors: symptoms such as nausea that could be indicative of ketosis

Blood or urine ketones should be checked whenever the blood glucose level is unexpectedly or repeatedly >250–300 mg/dL (>13.8–16.7 mmol/L). The same is true during intercurrent illness, especially a gastrointestinal illness, regardless of the blood glucose concentration. Illness can trigger diabetic ketoacidosis, thus, rapid identification and intervention can prevent severe illness and possible hospitalization. In addition, ketosis can cause nausea, vomiting, and abdominal pain. Because of the increased risk for euglycemic ketoacidosis associated with SGLT inhibitors, it is especially important to remind patients on these agents to check their ketone levels. Even if their glucose is normal, the development of any symptoms, such as nausea, could be indicative of ketosis.

For patients using an insulin pump, ketones should be measured whenever they experience "unexplained" hyperglycemia. In this setting, the presence of ketonuria or ketonemia may indicate failure of the insulin delivery system. Urinary ketones should be monitored daily in women who are pregnant.

MONITORING BY THE HEALTH-CARE TEAM

Overall metabolic control in people with diabetes is assessed primarily by four factors:

- Average overall blood glucose and A1C levels
- Frequency and severity of hypoglycemia
- Adequacy of growth, weight gain, and physical development in children and weight in adults
- Plasma lipid levels

At the outset of intensive diabetes management, after daily to weekly office visits when the program is being implemented and adjusted, the patient will require scheduled visits to assess the success of the program (see Table 8.2).

Table 8.2—Monitoring Metabolic Control

- Routinely determine A1C (estimated average glucose)
- Review SMBG results carefully at every visit, as well as between visits (if necessary)
- Review the frequency, severity, recognition, and treatment of hypoglycemia
- Assess growth, weight gain, and physical development in children and adolescents and weight in adults
- Take a careful history related to the management of sick days and occurrence of keto-acidosis
- Review issues of diet, including weight, and any difficulties in adherence to the overall management plan
- Monitor blood lipids annually

It is common practice to assess a patient's glycemic control and general health status quarterly. This schedule usually is sufficient for the patient using intensive diabetes management after the initial phase of stabilization. At each visit,

- measure A1C;
- check accuracy of blood glucose monitoring;
- review blood glucose data;
- study problems with hypoglycemia;
- identify and discuss any barriers to intensive diabetes management;
- discuss issues of diet;
- note body weight, blood pressure, and growth and physical development in children; and
- examine sites of insulin administration.

A1C—ESTIMATED AVERAGE GLUCOSE

The A1C test reflects mean glycemia over the preceding 2–3 months and is an essential component of diabetes management. The A1C should be measured at least twice a year in patients who are meeting treatment goals and quarterly in patients whose therapy has changed or who are not at goal. Monthly A1C measurements may be useful during periods of changing diabetes regimens. Converting A1C measurements into an estimated average glucose value translates the A1C into a number that patients can understand more readily and may make treatment goals more tangible (see Table 8.3). Individual variations in the rate of hemoglobin glycation, however, can contribute to inaccuracy in estimating the average glucose from A1C levels, and it is important for clinicians to inform patients about this uncertainty.

A1C can be measured by several different methods. The International Federation of Clinical Chemistry and Laboratory Medicine (IFCC) recently developed a method that specifically measures the concentration of one molecular species of A1C. This new IFCC method allows for worldwide standardization of A1C measurements performed using different methodologies. Adoption of this new reference standard will facilitate direct comparison of A1C measurements from different laboratories and will ensure the accuracy of the A1C-derived average glucose measurements used for clinical care.

Table 8.3—Correlation between A1C Level and Estimated Average Glucose Level

A1C (%)	Glucose Level	
	mg/dL (95% CIs)	mmol/L
6	126 (100–152)	7.0 (5.5– 8.5)
7	154 (123–185)	8.6 (6.8–10.3)
8	183 (147–217)	10.2 (8.1–12.1)
9	212 (170–249)	11.8 (9.4–13.9)
10	240 (193–282)	13.4 (10.7–15.7)
11	269 (217–314)	14.9 (12.0–17.5)
12	298 (240–347)	16.5 (13.3–19.3)

MONITORING FOR LONG-TERM COMPLICATIONS

The long-term complications of diabetes include retinopathy and cataracts; renal insufficiency and hypertension; autonomic and peripheral neuropathy; and macrovascular disease manifested by myocardial infarction, stroke, and peripheral vascular disease. Although improved glycemic control, with intensive diabetes therapy, delays the onset and slows the progression of retinopathy, nephropathy, and neuropathy and improves the risk factor profile related to macrovascular disease, complications of diabetes have not yet been eliminated. Therefore, monitoring for their presence and appropriate intervention or referral to appropriate specialists are required (see Table 8.4).

Table 8.4—Monitoring for Long-Term Complications

- Comprehensive annual dilated eye and visual examination, beginning
  - when diagnosed with type 2 diabetes
  - duration of type 1 diabetes of 5 years (and ≥10 years old)
  - age >30 years, regardless of duration
  - any visual symptoms or abnormalities
- Monitor blood lipids annually
- Careful examination of the feet (sensation, pulses, reflexes) at each visit
- Careful assessment of blood pressure at each visit
- Annual determination of urinary albumin after diabetes duration >5 years (patients with type 1 diabetes); children ≥10 years old; at diagnosis and annually thereafter (patients with type 2 diabetes)
- Monitor serum creatinine annually for determination of estimated *glomerular filtration rate* (eGFR) in all adults regardless of urine albumin excretion

RETINAL EXAMINATIONS

A comprehensive examination by an optometrist or ophthalmologist is recommended for all patients with type 2 diabetes (T2D) at the time of diagnosis, for all patients with type 1 diabetes (T1D) within 5 years after diagnosis, and for any patient with diabetes who has visual symptoms or abnormalities. Subsequent examinations should be repeated at least annually, or more frequently if advanced retinopathy is noted. Women who are planning pregnancy or who are pregnant also should have a comprehensive eye examination and require ophthalmologic follow-up throughout pregnancy.

Retinopathy initially may worsen during the first months of intensive diabetes management. This worsening is more often reported in patients who have poor glycemic control and more advanced retinopathy before the initiation of intensive therapy. In the DCCT, retinopathy progression was greater in the intensively treated cohort at the end of the first year. By the end of the second year, this difference was not significant, and thereafter the intensively treated cohort had a lower rate of retinopathy progression. Therefore, any patients undertaking intensive management should have a retinal examination before beginning intensive management and should discuss the plans for intensive management with their eye care professional, especially if metabolic control has been poor.

LIPID SCREENING

Lipid abnormalities play an important role in macrovascular disease. In recognition of this, diabetes is regarded as a risk factor for cardiovascular events equivalent to a previous cardiac event. In adults, a screening lipid profile should be performed at the time of first diagnosis, at the initial medical evaluation, or at age 40 years and periodically (e.g., every 1–2 years) thereafter. The profile should be assessed more often in patients with abnormal lipid values or inadequate blood glucose control. Abnormal lipid values should trigger intervention, including dietary and exercise counseling, attempts to achieve better glycemic control, and lipid-lowering medication, as indicated. To estimate risk for atherosclerotic cardiovascular disease (CVD), the American College of Cardiology/American Heart Association's Risk Calculator (http://my.americanheart.org) is a valuable tool in therapeutic decision making.

BLOOD PRESSURE

Blood pressure should be measured at each visit. If it is elevated, repeated measures should be taken to confirm the presence of hypertension, and antihypertensive therapy should be implemented. Most epidemiological studies have suggested that risk caused by elevated blood pressure is a continuous function; therefore, blood pressure cutoff levels are arbitrary. A recent large-scale intervention study suggests that lowering the systolic blood pressure to <120 mmHg can reduce risk for cardiac events, stroke, or death. In children, blood pressure should be decreased to the corresponding age, gender, and height-adjusted 90th percentile values.

URINARY ALBUMIN SCREENING

Measurement of urinary albumin excretion should be performed annually in all individuals ≥10 years old with T1D duration of at least 5 years. Because of the difficulty in precisely dating the onset of T2D, such screening should begin at the time of diagnosis in adults and in children who have type 2 diabetes. Screening for albuminuria can be performed by measuring the albumin-to-creatinine ratio in a random, spot urine collection. Screening may be confounded by orthostatic proteinuria; therefore, abnormal results should be repeated on first morning urine specimens.

FOOT EXAMINATIONS

Patients should have an annual foot examination to identify high-risk foot conditions related to diabetes. The examination should include inspection to assess hygiene and to determine the presence of any ulcers or infection. The assessment also should include a careful history to ascertain the presence of numbness, paresthesiae (tingling), or weakness. Pulses should be palpated, and reflexes and sensation should be checked. Individuals who have reduced sensation or pulses, foot deformities, or callus formation should have a careful foot examination at each routine office visit.

BIBLIOGRAPHY

American Diabetes Association. Preventive foot care in people with diabetes (Position Statement). *Diabetes Care* 2004;27(Suppl. 1):S63–S64

American Diabetes Association. Standards of medical care in diabetes—2016. *Diabetes Care* 2016;39(Suppl. 1):S1–S111

American Diabetes Association, European Association for the Study of Diabetes, International Federation of Clinical Chemistry and Laboratory Medicine, and the International Diabetes Federation. Consensus statement on the worldwide standardization of hemoglobin A1C measurement. *Diabetes Care* 2007;30:2399–2400

Fong DS, Aiello LP, Ferris FL III, Klein R. Diabetic retinopathy. *Diabetes Care* 2004;27:2540–2553

Nathan DM, Kuenen J, Borg R, Zheng H, Schoenfeld D, Heine R. Translating the A1c assay into estimated average glucose values. *Diabetes Care* 2008;31:1–6

Rosenstock J, Ferrannini E. Euglycemic diabetic ketoacidosis: a predictable, detectable, and preventable safety concern with SGLT2 inhibitors. *Diabetes Care* 2015;38:1638–1642

Wilson DM, Xing D, Cheng J, Beck RW, Hirsch I, Kollman C, Laffel L, Lawrence JM, Mauras N, Ruedy K, Tsalikian E, Wolpert H. Juvenile Diabetes Research Foundation Continuous Glucose Monitoring Study Group: persistence of individual variations in glycated hemoglobin. *Diabetes Care* 2011;34:1315–1317

Nutrition Management

DOI: 10.2337/9781580406321.09

Highlights
Nutrition Management

- Medical nutrition therapy (MNT) is integral to the implementation of all intensified forms of diabetes care.

- The primary goals of MNT are to promote metabolic control (including near-normal blood glucose and lipid levels), blood pressure control, and appropriate weight management. The nutrition plan must also prevent, or at least slow, the development of long-term diabetes complications, address individual nutrition needs (taking into account personal preferences and willingness to change), and promote pleasurable eating.

- MNT is often the most challenging aspect of diabetes management, leading to the recommendation that every person with diabetes regularly consult a registered dietitian knowledgeable about diabetes for development and periodic reevaluation of a personalized meal plan. Outcome studies demonstrate that MNT provided by registered dietitians can result in a 1–2% decrease in glycated hemoglobin A_{1c}.

- Target nutrition recommendations:
  - Urge development of a personalized plan based on an individual assessment.
  - Emphasize total carbohydrate intake as the primary nutrition factor affecting postprandial blood glucose levels, but also consider the type of carbohydrate ingested and the fat and protein contents of the meal.
  - Emphasize the role of weight loss in type 2 diabetes as a strategy to decrease insulin resistance and achieve glycemic and metabolic control.

- In type 1 diabetes, the meal plan should be based on the patient's usual intake with respect to calories, food selection, and meal timing. The insulin regimen should be fitted to the meal plan and adjusted based on the results of glucose monitoring.

- In type 2 diabetes, the dietitian should review the patient's usual intake and advise the patient to distribute calories and carbohydrates throughout the day, avoiding large concentrations at any one time. If the patient is overweight, a moderate calorie restriction (250–500 kcal/day) should be recommended, in concert with advice regarding physical activity and other behavioral or lifestyle modifications, as needed.

- Carbohydrate counting is a meal-planning approach well suited to intensive diabetes management because it allows matching of mealtime insulin delivery to carbohydrate-related insulin requirement.

- Glucose monitoring is an essential component of all approaches to intensified diabetes management. The joint evaluation of food and glucose records is a powerful tool for glucose control, and it allows fine-tuning of both nutrition and medication treatment plans.

- Hypoglycemia is a significant risk of intensive management. Nutrition factors often play a role in the cause and prevention of hypoglycemia.

- Greater precision in glucose control can be promoted through calibrated treatment of hypoglycemia, taking into account both the patient's dose response to oral glucose and the current and target glucose values.

- Weight gain may accompany intensive management when significant improvement in glucose control is achievedpotentially due to a reduction of glycosuria and/or consumption of extra calories to treat more frequent hypoglycemia. Strategies to prevent weight gain include reducing calories at the outset of intensive management, increasing physical activity, and rigorous MNT.

Nutrition Management

Medical nutrition therapy (MNT) is integral to successful diabetes management and is especially important for intensive diabetes management. Patients who use basal-bolus insulin regimens and frequent capillary blood glucose or continuous glucose monitoring (CGM) to maintain tight glucose control must apply sophisticated nutrition management skills to fully realize the potential of their intensive management plan. As demonstrated in the Diabetes Control and Complications Trial (DCCT), extensive, individual nutrition training and problem solving are required to support effective intensive management in patients with type 1 diabetes (T1D).

When considering intensifying the management of patients with type 2 diabetes (T2D), note that most patients with T2D receive little or no nutrition counseling before starting insulin therapy. Insulin initiation appears to be the most common factor that triggers primary care physicians to refer patients with T2D for nutrition counseling. Those patients who manage their diabetes with lifestyle modification or oral hypoglycemic agents or for whom nutrition is the primary or sole treatment modality are least likely to receive assistance with the nutrition component of their management. Extending MNT to this population would, in itself, represent a major "intensification" of their care.

GOALS OF MEDICAL NUTRITION THERAPY

The overall goal of MNT in diabetes care is to promote metabolic control. Included in this general objective are several specific targets (see Table 9.1). To achieve these goals, dietitians and other health-care professionals must educate people with diabetes to manage their nutrition intake in respect to a variety of individual factors, including medication, physical activity, illness and other stressors, and lifestyle considerations (e.g., work or school schedules; personal preferences; motivation; and economic, cultural, and religious concerns).

Consistent management and modification of food intake are often the most complex and challenging aspects of diabetes care. The complexity of these tasks is due to many factors (see Table 9.2). For this reason every person with prediabetes or diabetes should consult a registered dietitian (RD), preferably one familiar with the components of diabetes MNT, to obtain an individual nutrition plan. Because nutrition intake interacts with medication and physical activity in determining blood glucose levels, nutrition care must be fully integrated with other aspects of diabetes management to be effective. This is best accomplished through a team

Table 9.1—Goals of MNT Applicable to All Individuals with Diabetes

- Achieve and maintain the following:
  - Blood glucose levels in normal range or as close to normal as safely possible
  - Blood lipid and lipoprotein profiles that reduce risk for cardiovascular and peripheral vascular disease
  - Blood pressure levels in normal range or as close to normal as safely possible
- Prevent (or at least slow) rate of development of complications of diabetes
- Address individual nutrition needs, taking into account personal and cultural preferences and readiness, willingness, and ability to change
- Promote pleasurable eating, modifying food choices only if indicated by scientific evidence

approach. At a minimum, however, successful MNT requires open communication between the dietitian and other care providers. Furthermore, patients will likely benefit most from a series of encounters dedicated to nutrition education and problem solving to help develop the sophisticated skills required for successful management. Regular review and adjustment of the nutrition plan are also needed for optimal results.

TARGET NUTRITION RECOMMENDATIONS

The current nutrition principles and recommendations for diabetes, as formulated by the American Diabetes Association, focus on lifestyle goals and strategies for both the prevention and treatment of diabetes (see Table 9.3).

A personalized nutrition prescription should be based on individual assessment and should consider treatment goals and lifestyle changes the patient is willing and able to make. Clinical outcomes should be monitored and, if necessary, the nutrition prescription should be modified. This method has replaced specific guidelines for one "standard" diet or meal-planning method for all people with diabetes.

Table 9.2—Factors That Contribute to the Complexity of Nutrition Care

- Interaction of diabetes MNT with coexisting pathology (e.g., abnormal lipids, elevated blood pressure, and other health problems)
- Need to integrate MNT into other components of diabetes treatment regimen
- Need for advanced problem-solving skills to permit self-management
- Need for stepwise training to progressively build requisite knowledge and skills
- Inherent difficulty in modifying lifelong food behaviors and preferences
- Dynamic nature of both diabetes and life circumstances that demands periodic and creative modification of nutrition plan
- Need to meet all of these challenges while preserving patient autonomy and quality of life

Table 9.3 — Target Nutrition Recommendations for All People with Diabetes

Carbohydrate

- A dietary pattern that includes carbohydrate from fruits, vegetables, whole grains, legumes, and dairy products is encouraged for good health.
- Monitoring carbohydrate, whether by carbohydrate counting, or experience-based estimation, is a key strategy in achieving glycemic control.
- The use of the glycemic index and glycemic load may modestly improve glycemic control (at least when compared with considering total carbohydrate alone).
- Sucrose-containing foods can be substituted for other carbohydrates in the meal plan or, if added to the meal plan, can be covered with insulin or other glucose-lowering medications. Care should be taken to avoid excess energy intake and maintain nutritional balance.
- Sugar alcohols and nonnutritive sweeteners are safe when consumed within the daily intake levels established by the U.S. Food and Drug Administration.
- People with diabetes are encouraged to consume a variety of fiber-containing foods. There is no evidence, however, to recommend a higher fiber intake for people with diabetes than for the general population.

Protein

- For individuals with diabetes and normal renal function, evidence is insufficient to suggest that standard protein intake recommendations (15–20% of energy) should be modified.
- In individuals with T2D, ingested protein can increase insulin response without increasing plasma glucose concentrations. Therefore, protein should not be used to treat acute hypoglycemia or to prevent night time hypoglycemia.
- In individuals with T1D, ingested protein can increase blood glucose concentrations in the absence of sufficient active insulin. Individuals observing such an effect of dietary protein may benefit from education and adjustment of prandial insulin doses accordingly.
- The long-term effects of protein intake >20% of calories on diabetes management are unknown. Although such diets may produce short-term weight loss and improve glycemia, it has not been established that these benefits are maintained, and long-term effects on kidney function for people with diabetes are unknown.

Fat

- Evidence is inconclusive for an ideal amount of total fat intake for people with diabetes; therefore, goals should be individualized. Fat quality appears to be far more important than quantity.
  - In people with T2D, a Mediterranean-style diet, following a monounsaturated fatty acid–rich eating pattern, may be beneficial to glycemic control and may reduce risk factors for cardiovascular disease. This eating pattern may be an effective alternative to a lower-fat, higher-carbohydrate eating pattern.
  - Evidence does not support recommending omega-3 (EPA and DHA) supplements for people with diabetes for the prevention or treatment of cardiovascular events.
  - As recommended for the general public, an increase in foods containing long-chain omega-3 fatty acids (EPA and DHA) from fatty fish and omega-3 linolenic acid (ALA) is recommended for individuals with diabetes because of their beneficial effects on lipoproteins, prevention of heart disease, and associations with positive health outcomes in observational studies.

- The recommendation for the general public to eat fish (particularly fatty fish) at least two times (two servings) per week is also appropriate for people with diabetes.
- The amount of dietary saturated fat, cholesterol, and trans fat recommended for people with diabetes is the same as that recommended for the general population.
- In individuals with T1D, dietary fat can indirectly increase blood glucose concentrations in the absence of sufficient active insulin, primarily through increased acute insulin resistance and hepatic glucose output. Individuals observing such an effect of dietary fat may benefit from education and adjustment of prandial insulin doses accordingly.

Macronutrients

- The mix of carbohydrate, protein, and fat in the diet may be adjusted to meet the metabolic goals and individual preferences of people with diabetes.

Micronutrients

- There is no clear evidence of a benefit from vitamin or mineral supplementation in people with diabetes who do not have underlying deficiencies compared with the general population.
- Individual meal planning should include optimization of food choices to meet recommended daily allowance/dietary reference intake for all micronutrients.
- Routine supplementation with antioxidants, such as vitamins E and C and carotene, is not advised because of the lack of evidence of efficacy and concern related to long-term safety. B12 deficiency also can occur.
- Benefit from chromium supplementation in individuals with diabetes or obesity has not been clearly demonstrated and, therefore, cannot be recommended.

Alcohol

- If adults with diabetes choose to consume alcohol, daily intake should be limited to a moderate amount (one drink per day or less for adult women and two drinks per day or less for adult men). One drink is defined as 12 oz beer, 5 oz wine, or 1.5 oz ~80-proof spirits.
- Alcohol acutely impairs glucose release from the liver. To reduce the risk of hypoglycemia in individuals using insulin or insulin secretagogues, alcohol should be consumed with food and blood glucose levels monitored closely for 12–24 h.
- In individuals with diabetes, moderate consumption of alcohol may have a minimal effect on glucose and insulin concentrations, but when combined in carbohydrate-containing beverages—such as mixed drinks, sweet wines, and regular beer—it may raise blood glucose.

The recommendations acknowledge scientific evidence that sucrose and other simple sugars do not inherently impair diabetes control, opening the way for the inclusion of many traditionally "forbidden" foods in diabetes meal plans.

Modest weight loss (5% body weight) decreases insulin resistance in individuals with diabetes who are overweight or obese. The overarching goal for people with diabetes is to achieve blood glucose, blood pressure, and blood lipid levels in the normal range, or as close to normal as is safely possible, whether by weight loss or other means. Standardized diets and simplistic advice to "avoid sugar" and "lose weight," which have too often accounted for the totality of nutrition advice, are clearly inadequate. The current guidelines are compatible with a shift to more intensified programs of management for all people with diabetes. A flow chart describing the major steps in the design and implementation of meal plans consis-

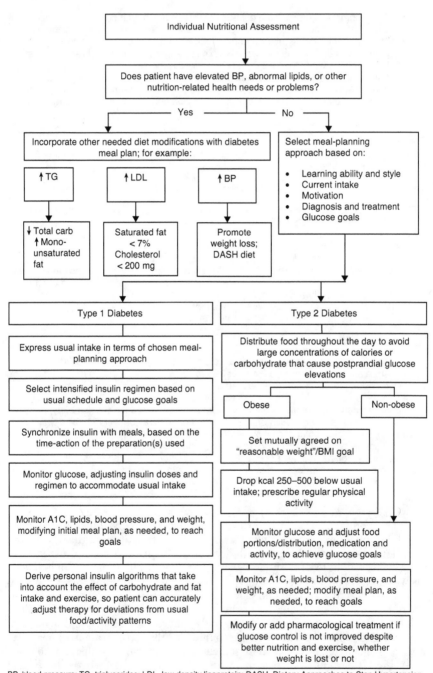

BP, blood pressure; TG, triglycerides; LDL, low density lipoprotein; DASH, Dietary Approaches to Stop Hypertension

Figure 9.1—Nutrition management flow chart.

Table 9.4—Integrating Recommendations Into the Nutrition Care Process

Implementation of MNT

- Upon diagnosis or first referral to a dietitian, 3–4 encounters lasting 45–90 min are recommended within 3–6 months.
- The dietitian should then determine whether additional MNT encounters are needed.
- At least 1 follow-up encounter annually is recommended to reinforce education or lifestyle changes, evaluate and monitor outcomes, and determine any need for change in MNT or medications. Dietitian should determine whether additional MNT encounters are needed.

Nutrition Assessment

- Client history, including medication and supplement history, past medical history, family history, and social history.
- Food and nutrition history, including food intake (composition, adequacy, meal or snack patterns, environmental cues to eating, tolerance, current diets or food modifications); nutrition health awareness and management (knowledge and beliefs about nutrition recommendations, self-monitoring and management practices, prior education); physical activity and exercise (functional status, activity patterns, sedentary time, exercise intensity, frequency, and duration); and food availability (food planning, purchasing, preparation abilities and limitations, food safety, food program utilization, food insecurity).
- Biochemical data, medical tests, and procedures, including laboratory data (A1C, lipid profile, kidney function).
- Anthropometric measurements, including height, weight, body mass index (BMI), growth rate, and rate of weight change.
- Nutrition-focused physical findings, including general physical appearance, body language, digestive system, and blood pressure.

Nutrition Intervention:

- Implement MNT, selecting from a variety of nutrition interventions to help patients achieve individualized nutrition goals.
- Encourage consumption of macronutrients based on dietary reference intakes for healthy children and adults.
- Implement nutrition education and counseling with emphasis on recommendations from major and contributing factors to nutrition therapy.

Nutrition Monitoring and Evaluation:

- Coordinate care with interdisciplinary team.
- Monitor and evaluate food intake, medication, metabolic control, anthropometric measurements, and physical activity.
- Use blood glucose monitoring results to evaluate achievement of goals and effectiveness of MNT. Glucose monitoring results can help determine whether food or medication need to be adjusted.

tent with the current recommendations is shown in Fig. 9.1. Some ways to integrate recommendations into the nutrition care process are listed in Table 9.4.

STRATEGIES FOR TYPE 1 DIABETES

The following strategies are the starting points for the nutrition component of intensified management for people with T1D. They form the basis of care, regardless of the specific meal-planning approach used.

- Insulin therapy should be integrated into an individual's dietary and physical activity pattern.
- Individuals using rapid-acting insulin, either by injection or insulin pump, should adjust meal and snack insulin doses based on the carbohydrate in their meals and snacks.
- Individuals using fixed daily insulin doses should keep daily carbohydrate intake consistent with respect to time and amount.
- For planned exercise, insulin doses can be adjusted. For unplanned exercise, extra carbohydrate may be needed.

Maintaining a consistent carbohydrate intake can be extremely challenging. On presentation, newly diagnosed individuals with T1D often have experienced weight loss and have an increase in appetite with the initiation of insulin therapy. Therefore, base the initial diabetes meal plan on the patient's appetite to restore or maintain appropriate body weight and allow for normal growth and development. Once the initial meal plan has been established, monitor weight, blood pressure, A1C, lipids, and other clinical parameters to determine whether further modifications are needed to meet goals.

For individuals using either multiple daily injections (MDI) or continuous subcutaneous insulin infusion (CSII), lifestyle flexibility and maintaining optimal blood glucose control is achieved by developing personal algorithms that take into account the interplay of insulin, food intake, and physical activity. Using these algorithms, patients are able to systematically adjust therapy as needed in response to deviations from usual patterns.

Two different approaches can be used when a patient initiates intensive diabetes management. The first approach is a fixed carbohydrate and insulin plan, which involves prescribing a consistent carbohydrate meal plan based on the patient's usual intake and nutrition requirements. Prandial insulin dosages are then adjusted to the amount of carbohydrate in each meal to achieve target glycemia levels. Once the optimal insulin dosage for each meal is established, the insulin dose is "fixed." Education around the amount of carbohydrate in different foods should be provided, so that the source of carbohydrate (e.g., fruit versus dairy versus grains) can be varied without changing the total carbohydrate content of the meal or snack.

For patients who are skilled in carbohydrate counting and desiring the flexibility of eating varying amounts of carbohydrate, a second approach is useful, namely, a flexible carbohydrate and insulin plan. This approach prescribes an insulin dose per quantity of carbohydrate (insulin-to-carbohydrate ratio), so that the prandial insulin dose can be adjusted based on the desired amount of carbohydrate in the meal. For example, if a patient has an insulin-to-carbohydrate ratio of 1:10 g and wants to eat 50 g of carbohydrate, they will then require 5 units of insulin (50 divided by 10). This approach allows patients more flexibility with food choices and quantities. The insulin-to-carbohydrate ratio can be determined based on experience or the Rule of 500. For example, if a patient consistently eats a lunch containing about 72 g of carbohydrate and requires 8 units of rapid-acting insulin when the prelunch blood glucose level is at target, this patient requires 1 unit of insulin for every 9 g of carbohydrate at lunch (72 divided by 8).

For patients skilled in carbohydrate counting but who have difficulty eating consistent amounts of carbohydrate, a second approach uses a formula to determine the insulin-to-carbohydrate ratio. This approach is known as the equal to 500 divided by the total daily insulin dose. For example, a patient whose total daily insulin dose is 50 units would divide 500 by 50 to achieve a ratio of 1:10. This ratio then may need to be adjusted (fine-tuned) based on an evaluation of postprandial blood glucose levels and food records. It is common for patients to have different insulin-to-carbohydrate ratios for different meals.

These meal-planning strategies arise from a strong scientific and behavioral base and describe a much less prescriptive approach than commonly has been used in the past. They acknowledge the difficulty in changing ingrained food habits, the wide range of diets that can be compatible with good diabetes control, and the importance of prioritizing the patient's preferences and lifestyle values while supporting increased flexibility and patient choice to the overall plan of care. Like other aspects of intensified management, they require more time and skill on the part of health-care providers and patients than do more traditional approaches.

STRATEGIES FOR TYPE 2 DIABETES

For patients with T2D, the primary focus of MNT is on weight loss and lifestyle strategies to improve abnormalities in glucose, lipid, and blood pressure and to reduce the risk of chronic complications, especially cardiovascular disease. Near-normal blood glucose control reduces insulin resistance and preserves insulin secretory capacity in T2D. Hypocaloric diets and modest weight loss (5–7% of body weight) often improve glycemic control in the short-term and, if maintained, can contribute to long-term improvements in glycemic control. Modest weight loss has been shown to improve insulin resistance in overweight (BMI ≥ 25 kg/m^2) and obese (BMI ≥ 30 kg/m^2) insulin-resistant individuals. The risk of comorbidity increases with BMIs in this range and higher. Waist circumference is used as a measure of visceral fat. A waist circumference of ≥ 35 inches in women and ≥ 40 inches in men is used in conjunction with BMI to assess the risk of cardiovascular disease as well as the risk for T2D.

Unfortunately, generally effective strategies for long-term maintenance of weight loss are unknown, and long-term weight loss is difficult for most people to achieve. Low-carbohydrate or low-fat calorie-restricted diets may be effective for weight loss in the short term (up to 1 year). Physical activity and behavior modification are important components of weight-loss programs and are adjuncts to MNT in maintaining weight loss.

A structured, intensive lifestyle program that encompasses education, counseling, behavioral therapy, reduced calorie and fat (<30% of total calories) intake, regular and sustained physical activity, and frequent contact with health-care providers is required to achieve a 5–7% weight loss. Physical activity alone has only a modest effect on weight loss, but nevertheless is important for improving insulin sensitivity, lowering blood glucose levels, and maintaining long-term weight loss. A weight loss plan of 500–1,000 fewer calories per week initially will result in a loss of ~1–2 pounds per week. Without continued support and follow-up, however, the weight is often regained.

Traditionally, low-fat diets have been prescribed for overweight or obese people with T2D. Because weight loss is difficult to sustain, other approaches recently have been explored, including low-carbohydrate diets. Evidence suggests that very low-carbohydrate diets, in the short term, may result in more weight loss than low-fat diets. In the longer term, however, differences in weight loss between very low-carbohydrate and low-fat diets are not significant, and weight loss is modest with both dietary approaches. The long-term effects of very low-carbohydrate diets are unknown; these diets may be deficient in fiber, vitamins, and minerals and usually rate low on palatability, thus making them difficult to sustain for a long period of time. A moderate reduction in carbohydrate can be considered for people with T2D and may be more efficacious.

Meal replacements are another dietary approach that may be considered for the overweight or obese patient with T2D. Meal replacements, typically consisting of shakes or prepackaged meals, can be safely used for one or two meals per day. They provide a defined amount of calories and nutrients and can result in significant weight loss. Use of meal replacements generally must be continued, however, to sustain the weight loss.

Conversely, very low-calorie diets (VLCDs) that provide ≤800 calories per day typically are not recommended as a weight-loss approach, despite the fact that they do result in significant weight loss and improved glycemic and lipid control. Long-term use of VLCD can be detrimental to good health and, when VLCDs are discontinued, weight is quickly regained. If a VLCD is considered, it must be part of a structured program that provides ongoing support.

Weight-loss medications have been used in combination with lifestyle changes to successfully promote weight loss (5–10%) among overweight or obese individuals with T2D. Pharmacological therapy for obesity should be used only in patients with a BMI >27 kg/m². For individuals with a BMI ≥35 kg/m², bariatric surgery has been shown to be an effective weight-loss treatment that can result in marked improvement in glycemia and cardiovascular risk factors, with the exception of hypercholesterolemia. The risks of bariatric surgery are serious and may include increased mortality, blood clots, hernia, infection, and dumping syndrome.

The following strategies form the basis for dietary intervention in all people with T2D. When applied in conjunction with active monitoring of glucose, they also delineate the nutrition component of intensified management for this group.

- The nutrition prescription should be based on lifestyle changes that patients are willing and able to make.
- Review the patient's usual intake with respect to total energy, food, and carbohydrate distribution throughout the day, fat intake (type and amount), and food selection.

- Distribute food throughout the day to eliminate large concentrations of calories or carbohydrate that may contribute to postprandial glucose elevation.
- Make recommendations regarding improvements in food choices to create a nutritionally adequate meal plan with reduced total, saturated, and trans fat, if needed.
- Advise patients regarding cholesterol intake per guidelines (see Table 9.3).
- If the patient is overweight, recommend moderate calorie restriction (no more than 250–500 kcal/day below estimated energy requirements) and regular physical activity to help promote modest, gradual weight loss. Calorie restriction is a valuable glucose control strategy for many people with T2D, whether or not weight loss is achieved.
- Monitor blood glucose and adjust food distribution, portions, and selection (as needed) in concert with medications and physical activity, to achieve glucose goals.
- Monitor weight, blood pressure, A1C, lipids, and other clinical parameters and modify the initial meal plan as needed to meet goals.

Traditionally defined "desirable" or "ideal" body weight is no longer used in setting weight goals for patients with diabetes. The guideline terminology "reasonable weight" refers to the weight an individual and his or her health-care provider agree can be achieved and maintained, in both the short and long term. In addition, goals for BMI and waist circumference, mutually agreed on by the patient and practitioner, may be more achievable and realistic than focusing on a predetermined body weight goal.

For overweight people with T2D, modest weight loss (10–15 lb or 5–7 kg), regardless of starting weight, often is associated with significant improvements in glycemic, lipid, and blood pressure control. Improved glycemia is more likely to occur relatively early in the course of diabetes when patients still have the capacity to produce effective levels of endogenous insulin. Patients who do not experience an improvement in glucose control with modest weight loss are unlikely to see any beneficial effect on glucose control with additional weight loss alone. Persistent fasting hyperglycemia despite a 10-lb (5-kg) weight loss suggests the need for initiation of, or changes in, pharmacological therapy. For patients with T2D using a basal-bolus insulin therapy, fixed or flexible carbohydrate intake and insulin doses (as described in the previous section) may be appropriate to match rapid-acting insulin to carbohydrate intake and optimize glycemia.

GLUCOSE MONITORING AND THE NUTRITION PLAN

BLOOD GLUCOSE MONITORING

Appropriate use of the results of blood glucose monitoring plays an essential role in the nutrition aspects of intensive diabetes management. Blood glucose monitoring provides the feedback needed to fine-tune the meal plan in concert with physical activity, medications (if used), and other relevant factors.

When evaluated in relation to food records, blood glucose monitoring can be used to refine the dietary approach in various ways. Postprandial glucose values can guide modification of the basic meal plan or can be used to tailor the patient's insulin-to-carbohydrate ratio or insulin adjustment algorithm. Review of food records in conjunction with glucose results reveals the effect of various single foods and food combinations. Such information, when used as the basis for determining prandial insulin dosing, can increase the patient's flexibility in food choices while maintaining or improving glucose control. Some sample monitoring strategies that help to fine-tune nutritional care are outlined in Table 9.5.

For all patients with T1D or T2D, the primary goal of MNT is to establish a healthy eating plan, using the principles of MNT previously described. If pre- or postprandial glucose values are not within the targeted range despite a healthy, balanced diet, it may be prudent to commence or adjust an oral medication, incretin mimetic, or insulin. Figure 9.1 illustrates schematically the process of nutrition intervention in intensive management, including the essential role of blood glucose monitoring in evaluating and adjusting intervention.

CONTINUOUS GLUCOSE MONITORING

Real-time continuous glucose monitoring (RT-CGM) systems use a subcutaneous glucose sensor to continually measure interstitial glucose concentrations. These systems provide detailed information on glucose patterns and trends, including postprandial glucose values that are difficult to ascertain by episodic monitoring of blood glucose concentrations. They also provide information on the direction and rate of change of glucose concentrations. By allowing patients to observe glucose values and trends as they occur, RT-CGM provides the patient with the opportunity to make decisions based on real-time glucose values and perform more timely therapy adjustments.

The data obtained from RT-CGM also allow for greater precision in matching the dose and timing of mealtime insulin to postprandial glucose profiles. RT-CGM can be especially helpful for adjusting the insulin dose for meals that produce complex postmeal glucose profiles (e.g., pizza). RT-CGM can be used to identify a problematic postmeal glucose pattern and then to monitor the postprandial pattern following various corrective bolusing schemes. In this way, the optimal dose and time parameters for the meal bolus can be determined.

RT-CGM data can be an important tool for reshaping eating behavior as patients receive immediate feedback on their personal glycemic responses to their food choices. RT-CGM has made it possible for users to more clearly see that the food factors that determine the postprandial glucose profile include not only the amount of carbohydrate but also the type of carbohydrate (i.e., glycemic index value) and the effect of fat, protein, caffeine, and alcohol. Foods with a high glycemic index may cause a postprandial glucose spike because of a mismatch between the rapid absorption of the carbohydrate and the less rapid onset of action of the insulin bolus. Protein can increase postprandial glucose levels through increased hepatic glucose output, although it is usually a delayed effect seen ~1.5 h after the meal. Fat can affect postprandial glucose levels by slowing gastric emptying, thereby delaying the increase in postmeal glucose levels and also by decreasing postprandial insulin sensitivity, leading to higher postmeal glucose levels than would be produced by a carbohydrate-equivalent low-fat meal. Caffeine, like fat, can reduce insulin sensitivity in some people, also leading to higher glucose levels.

Table 9.5—Using Blood Glucose Monitoring to Fine-Tune Nutrition Therapy

Type of Diabetes	Pharmacological Management	Blood Glucose Monitoring Schedule	Question to Ask	Strategy to Correct Elevated Blood Glucose
Type 2, obese	None; oral diabetes medication(s), incretin mimetic, or insulin	Fasting	Does the overnight insulin or other oral glucose-lowering agent suppress hepatic glucose output sufficiently to produce desired fasting blood glucose level?	Reduce total calories; review bedtime snack and any other foods eaten overnight. Evaluate pharmacological management.
		2- to 4-h postprandial or next pre-meal blood glucose	Does available insulin (endogenous or exogenous) cover the meal eaten, producing the desired postprandial value?	Reduce calories and/or carbohydrate/fat in meal. When obesity is present, food reduction and/or increased physical activity are preferred to increases in medication whenever possible. Consider the glycemic impact of carbohydrate ingested.
Type 1 or Type 2, non-obese	Insulin	Fasting	Does overnight exogenous insulin suppress hepatic glucose output sufficiently to produce desired fasting blood glucose level?	Adjust dose or timing of overnight insulin; review evening meal, bedtime snack, and any other foods eaten overnight. Consider adding another oral glucose-lowering agent or an incretin mimetic in patients with type 2 diabetes. Insulin coverage may be needed for bedtime snack in those patients on CSII or MDI therapy.
		2–4-h postprandial (rapid-acting insulin analog) or next pre-meal value (regular insulin)	Is the pre-meal insulin dose appropriate?	Adjust dose or timing of premeal insulin; fine-tune patient's insulin algorithm; evaluate impact of quantity of carbohydrate (and glycemic impact [GI/GL]) of carbohydrate), protein, or fat consumed.
		Pre-meal (CSII or MDI only)	Is the basal insulin dose or rate (CSII) correct?	Adjust basal insulin to bring premeal blood glucose into target range.

CSII, continuous subcutaneous insulin infusion; MDI, multiple dose injection; GI/GL, [AU: Please give full form.]

Alcohol has a glucose-lowering effect, as it blocks glucose release from the liver. Alcoholic beverages containing significant carbohydrate initially may cause an increase followed by a later decrease in glucose levels. The multiplicity of food factors affecting postprandial glucose levels can make diabetes control challenging for the patient. By providing feedback on glycemic responses to various food factors, RT-CGM can enable the motivated patient to improve glycemic control with less frequent hypoglycemia.

Having RT-CGM does not relieve the user of the need to perform blood glucose monitoring with use of a conventional blood glucose meter. All RT-CGM systems currently approved for patient use require calibration using a conventional blood glucose meter. Confirmation using a blood glucose meter is required before interstitial glucose values are used for immediate treatment decisions. Nevertheless, retrospective review of interstitial glucose values may be used to revise insulin dosing patterns.

HYPOGLYCEMIA

Nutrition strategies are important for the prevention of hypoglycemia in all people whose diabetes treatment includes insulin or an insulin secretagogue. Common nutrition factors that contribute to hypoglycemia risk are listed in Table 9.6; issues and strategies relative to each factor are discussed in the following sections.

OMITTING OR DELAYING PLANNED MEALS OR SNACKS

The risk of hypoglycemia from omitting or delaying meals is greatest in patients who use insulin regimens that include intermediate- and short-acting (regular) insulin. The increased risk is attributable to high circulating insulin levels between meals and overnight owing to the time–action profiles of intermediate- and short-acting insulin. The risk of hypoglycemia also may be high if meals or snacks are omitted or delayed in patients using MDI regimens or in patients using an insulin secretagogue. Patients whose diabetes is treated by diet alone or those who use oral glucose-lowering agents, such as biguanides, pioglitazone, or dipeptidyl peptidase-IV inhibitors (DPP-IV), as monotherapy are not at increased risk of hypoglycemia when meals are delayed or omitted.

Table 9.6—Nutrition Factors Contributing to Hypoglycemia

- Omitting or delaying planned meals or snacks
- Inappropriate timing of meals relative to insulin
- Imbalance between food and meal-related insulin dose because of
  - inaccurate estimation of carbohydrate intake when calculating meal-related boluses
  - consuming less carbohydrate than usual without adjusting insulin dose
- Inadequate carbohydrate supplementation for physical activity
- Consuming alcohol without food (or without adjusting insulin dose)
- Delayed absorption of carbohydrate when eating high-fat or low-glycemic-index meals and using a rapid-acting insulin analog

The risk for hypoglycemia should be considered when selecting a pharmacological regimen. Individuals whose work or other activities make it difficult to predict or control mealtimes (e.g., trial lawyers, inpatient medical staff, traveling salespeople) will have less frequent hypoglycemia using insulin regimens that allow more mealtime flexibility.

All patients whose diabetes treatment includes insulin or an insulin secretagogue should receive education regarding appropriate meal timing for their particular regimen. Carrying a source of rapidly absorbed carbohydrate is a vital self-management behavior for all such patients to prevent hypoglycemia, particularly when meals are unavoidably delayed.

INAPPROPRIATE TIMING OF INSULIN RELATIVE TO MEALS

The risk for hypoglycemia is greatest when the peak action of insulin is not synchronized with the peak of glucose entry into the bloodstream after a meal. Consider the following common scenario: the patient takes a bolus of short-acting insulin immediately before eating. Hyperglycemia occurs in the immediate postprandial period, because carbohydrate is absorbed but insulin has not yet reached its peak action. Two to three hours later, when little or no carbohydrate is entering the circulation and insulin action has reached its peak, blood glucose levels decrease and hypoglycemia may occur. Delaying the meal results in a better match between insulin action and postprandial glucose availability, but this solution is difficult for many patients to implement. Rapid-acting insulin analogs (lispro, aspart, glulisine), which achieve their peak action earlier than regular insulin, shorten the interval between administering the bolus and eating the meal. The shorter total duration of action of these insulins also reduces the risk for between-meal and nocturnal hypoglycemia. When intermediate-acting insulin is injected in the morning, it is necessary to schedule lunch at the time when this insulin is peaking to reduce the risk of prelunch hypoglycemia. Blood glucose monitoring should be used to confirm optional insulin timing relative to meals because the action profiles of specific insulin preparations vary considerably from person to person and also are affected by injection site, exercise, and other factors.

In addition to modifying insulin administration or meal timing, another strategy to reduce the risk for hypoglycemia between meals is to include snacks in the meal plan. Snacks often are needed to prevent hypoglycemia in individuals using premixed insulins (see Chapter 6) because of the broad peak action curves of short-acting and intermediate-acting insulin (NPH insulin). The need for snacks often can be eliminated by using rapid-acting insulin analogs in combination with a long-acting insulin, either glargine or detemir, to provide between-meal insulin coverage.

IMBALANCE BETWEEN FOOD AND MEAL-RELATED INSULIN DOSE

Hypoglycemia may result when the meal-related insulin dose is too large relative to the amount of food eaten. In the intensively managed MDI or CSII patient who adjusts premeal boluses for anticipated intake, hypoglycemia most often occurs because of errors in estimating food or carbohydrate intake. Bolus calculations can be based on carbohydrate choices, carbohydrate intake, or known meal composition, but irrespective of the method used, the algorithm used must be individualized to the patient. Most people benefit from a period of weighing and measuring their food to train their eye to accurately estimate portion sizes.

Unless the blood glucose level is decreasing rapidly, the meal insulin bolus should be given before starting the meal. In special circumstances, it may be advisable to inject the meal bolus at the end of a meal. Doing so allows more calibration of the bolus to the actual amount eaten and is particularly helpful in the management of young children with diabetes and during illness or pregnancy, when nausea may interfere with eating.

For patients on a fixed insulin plan, a fixed meal plan is required. If one parameter changes, the other must reflect this change. Although not all patients will choose to increase insulin doses to accommodate extra food intake—perhaps as a means of weight management—they should at least be given instruction on how to prevent hypoglycemia if a smaller-than-normal meal is eaten. Individual guidelines for insulin reduction could be used, or the missing carbohydrate could be replaced with another equivalent carbohydrate source, such as fruit or a snack.

INADEQUATE FOOD SUPPLEMENTATION FOR EXERCISE

Blood glucose monitoring is required to calibrate insulin doses or carbohydrate intake to reduce hypoglycemia risk with exercise. The decision whether to adjust food or insulin is determined by the individual's diabetes management goals and is affected by whether the exercise is planned. When exercise is planned, the dose of insulin acting during the period of physical activity can be reduced to minimize hypoglycemia risk (see Chapter 6).

If exercise is not planned with sufficient time to permit insulin dose adjustment, additional carbohydrate usually is needed to prevent exercise-related hypoglycemia. Depending on the blood glucose level at the start of exercise, as well as the intensity and duration of the activity, the extra carbohydrate may be taken before, during, or after exercise. If blood glucose levels are <100 mg/dL before starting exercise, carbohydrate should be ingested before the activity begins. During exercise of moderate intensity, glucose uptake is increased by 2–3 mg/kg/min or ~8–13 g/h, which supports the general recommendation to add 15 g carbohydrate for every 30–60 min of activity exceeding the patient's usual level of physical activity. Patients will need personalized guidelines based on blood glucose monitoring to guide carbohydrate supplementation for exercise. When exercise has been intense or prolonged, the risk for hypoglycemia extends up to 24 h postexercise. Therefore, additional snacks may be needed in the hours after exercise, or before bedtime, when strenuous exercise has occurred in the afternoon or evening. In addition, reduction of the amount of insulin administered after particularly lengthy or intense exercise may be required.

Exercise is a central component of overall diabetes management for individuals attempting to reach and maintain a reasonable body weight. It is obviously preferable to avoid increasing food intake to cover exercise in such individuals. To better support weight management and calorie restriction goals, exercise can be scheduled after meals when blood glucose levels are peaking. If exercising after meals is not possible, or if it does not prevent hypoglycemia, medication doses should be decreased to allow exercise to occur without having to increase food intake.

CONSUMING ALCOHOL ON AN EMPTY STOMACH

Alcohol inhibits gluconeogenesis and interferes with the counterregulatory response to insulin-induced hypoglycemia. Alcohol, therefore, may contribute to delayed hypoglycemia, especially in people with T1D. If sweet wines, liqueurs, or drinks made with regular soda or fruit juices are consumed, the carbohydrate may need to be offset with insulin. This should be done cautiously, however, because of the hypoglycemia risk associated with alcohol. Choosing dry wines, light beers, and drinks made with noncaloric mixers may simplify the management of alcohol consumption in people with diabetes who choose to consume alcohol. Checking the blood glucose level before going to sleep is a recommended safety precaution for patients who have been drinking alcohol. An extra bedtime snack or reduction in the dose of bedtime insulin may be necessary.

Because they typically are insulin resistant, alcohol-induced hypoglycemia is less of a risk in people with T2D, unless they are using insulin or an insulin secretagogue to manage their diabetes. Consuming alcohol with food can reduce the risk of hypoglycemia.

ORAL TREATMENT OF HYPOGLYCEMIA

Helping each patient develop a personally calibrated treatment plan for hypoglycemia is a valuable strategy to promote better blood glucose control. Overtreatment of hypoglycemia is common and often is caused by a lack of or inadequate advice on appropriate treatment of hypoglycemia. When the same "take 15–20 g of carbohydrate" advice is given to all patients, the result will be inadequate treatment in some and excessive treatment in others. The increase in blood glucose level produced by a given amount of carbohydrate varies from person to person, primarily as a result of differences in body size and insulin sensitivity. For example, a given quantity of carbohydrate generally will increase the blood glucose level more in a small person than it will in a larger person.

To develop an individual hypoglycemia treatment algorithm for a patient, begin with the estimate that each 5 g of glucose increases blood glucose ~20 mg/dL (1.1 mmol/L; an approximate value for a 150-lb [69-kg] person). With subsequent blood glucose monitoring, fine-tune this value, based on the patient's response to given amounts of glucose. For example, suppose a 100-lb (45-kg) woman finds that her blood glucose level is 40 mg/dL (2.2 mmol/L), and she wants to increase her blood glucose level by ~60 mg/dL (3.3 mmol/L) to 100 mg/dL (5.6 mmol/L). If she treats the hypoglycemia with a 15-g carbohydrate expecting that each 5-g carbohydrate will increase her blood glucose 20 mg/dL but instead her blood glucose increases to 145 mg/dL (8.0 mmol/L), this demonstrates that every 5 g of glucose increases her blood glucose by 35 mg/dL. The patient then can calibrate treatment of a subsequent episode of hypoglycemia based on the current blood glucose concentration and a personal blood glucose target. Providing the patient with an algorithm can avoid a potential source of treatment error because it eliminates the patient's need to perform calculations in a hypoglycemic state.

Virtually any nonfat source of carbohydrate (e.g., saltines, regular soda, fruit juice, nonfat milk) can be used to treat hypoglycemia; however, glucose is the most rapid-acting carbohydrate source. Commercially prepared products, such as glucose tablets and glucose gels, are higher in available glucose than other high-carbohydrate foods that contain sugars such as fructose, which are of no benefit in raising blood glucose levels and furthermore add to the calories consumed from the treatment of hypoglycemia. In addition, they offer the advantages of more precise glucose dosing and a more predictable glucose absorption from the buccal mucosa. They also are more easily portable and unlikely to serve as a snack, so they are more likely to be available when hypoglycemia occurs.

FACILITATING NUTRITION SELF-MANAGEMENT

Achieving optimal glycemic control requires that the patient successfully balance food intake, diabetes medications, and physical activity. Rigid or strict diets generally are not conducive to achieving glycemic control, as they are not individualized to the unique characteristics, preferences, and lifestyle of the patient. In addition, most people are unable to sustain a structured eating plan for any significant length of time. Each patient who uses an intensified management approach must receive the depth of education required to build nutrition self-management skills.

As previously described, this process begins with a nutrition assessment to enable the dietitian to tailor MNT to each patient's unique circumstances. The ensuing education process progresses from the mutual identification of specific goals through appropriate stepwise intervention and is guided throughout by an evaluation of the patient's knowledge and skill, as well as by clinical parameters. These processes of assessment and education are similar for every patient, regardless of the specific approach to diabetes meal planning used.

MEAL-PLANNING APPROACHES FOR INTENSIFIED MANAGEMENT

Several distinct meal-planning systems commonly are used in diabetes MNT. Each stresses a different factor (e.g., calories, portion control, food choices, fat, or carbohydrate content). The DCCT demonstrated that many different approaches to meal planning can be used successfully in intensive management regimens. The four major types of diabetes meal-planning systems and the benefits of each are summarized in Table 9.7. The choice of a specific meal-planning approach should be based on a review of the patient's current intake and food choices, clinical goals, learning style, and desire for flexibility.

Always consider the amount of time necessary to teach various meal-planning approaches. Sufficient and effective patient education and support materials must be available. Similarly, all approaches entail a staged program of education, progressing from simple concepts of diabetes nutrition management to the more in-depth knowledge that supports nutrition self-management and informed decision making.

Table 9.7 – Benefits and Drawbacks of Major Types of Meal-Planning Systems

System type	Description	Benefits	Drawbacks
General guidelines	USDA Choose My Plate Guidelines; Dietary Guidelines for Americans	Easy to understand Good initial teaching tools Focus is on healthy food choices	Low emphasis on measuring portions complicates coordinating insulin doses with food
Menu planning	Written-out individual sample menus	Specific Simple to use Can guide food choices while patient learns more advanced concepts Can use patient's preferred and available foods	Lack of flexibility to respond to unusual circumstances Keeps decision making in hands of caregiver instead of patient
Exchange/choice	Lists groups of foods of similar nutritional content, indicating portions of each that can be substituted for one another to provide variety; accompanied by a meal pattern that indicates the number of servings to be eaten from each group at each meal	Includes portion control Facilitates calorie adjustment Supports meal planning materials such as food lists, recipes, and menus Multiple nutrition concerns can be incorporated into a single plan	Exchange concept is difficult for many to understand Time-consuming to teach Can be limiting and prescriptive, especially if inadequate education is provided Does not always correlate with portions listed on food labels
Counting	Systems that focus on counting amounts of given nutrients: common ones are carbohydrate counting for glucose control and fat counting for calorie control or weight management	Allows greatest flexibility in food choices Emphasis is on carefully quantifying food intake Simple to teach and apply because of single-topic focus Carbohydrate counting is most common method for matching insulin to food intake	Other nutrition concepts (e.g., healthy food choices, cardiovascular risk reduction) must be taught separately Difficult for patients who are cognitively impaired or learning disabled

CARBOHYDRATE COUNTING

Carbohydrate counting is a meal planning system that involves determining the amount of carbohydrate eaten at a meal or a snack. Because dietary carbohydrate is the chief determinant of the meal-related insulin requirement, patients must be able to correctly identify the amount of carbohydrate in the meal for accurate insulin dosing. Patients can learn to count grams of carbohydrate or carbohydrate choices or exchanges, where one choice or exchange is equivalent to 10 or 15 g carbohydrate. Carbohydrate counting can be used as the sole meal-planning approach or in concert with other systems to fine-tune blood glucose control. The health-care provider also can use carbohydrate counting to determine the cause of unexplained blood glucose excursions.

Carbohydrate counting involves precisely counting the carbohydrate in a meal and then using an individual insulin-to-carbohydrate ratio to calculate the meal insulin dose. To determine the ratio of insulin needed for the amount of carbohydrate consumed, initially, basic carbohydrate counting can be implemented as a stable meal plan with a given quantity of carbohydrate for each meal and snack, preferably based on the patient's typical intake. During this initial period on a meal plan, the patient weighs and measures food portions (to gain skill in visually estimating portion sizes), reads food labels, and maintains complete food and blood glucose records. Evaluation of this data allows for the patient's insulin-to-carbohydrate ratio to be determined (i.e., the ratio between the grams of carbohydrate eaten and the number of units of mealtime insulin required). The insulin-to-carbohydrate ratio for adults with T1D is commonly in the range 1:10–1:15 (1 unit of insulin for each 10–15 g carbohydrate); however, this generalization cannot be made for every patient to optimize blood glucose control. The precise ratio for each patient is determined by reviewing food records and blood glucose monitoring results. For additional information on carbohydrate counting, refer to *Practical Carbohydrate Counting: A How-to-Teach Guide for Health Professionals* (see the Bibliography).

ADJUSTING INSULIN FOR PROTEIN AND FAT

Emerging evidence from recent research indicates that, in addition to carbohydrate, fat and protein can significantly modulate postprandial glucose concentrations in individuals with T1D. It is now recommended that selected individuals, who have mastered carbohydrate counting and are experiencing the glycemic impact of fat and protein, should receive education and adjust their mealtime insulin accordingly.

In the early postprandial period (first 2–3 h), dietary fat reduces the glycemic rise through delayed gastric emptying and can increase the potential for early hypoglycemia. Delayed gastric emptying can delay the peak postprandial glucose level. In the absence of sufficient insulin, meals containing a significant amount of dietary fat can cause substantial late postprandial hyperglycemia (>3 h) as acute insulin resistance and hepatic glucose output increases. High-fat meals can increase insulin requirements by more than twofold.

Likewise, protein can significantly increase late postprandial glycemia, although the effects differ depending on whether carbohydrate is included in the meal or not. When protein and carbohydrate are eaten together (e.g., sandwich with meat filling), as little as 30 g of protein can cause a significant increase in glycemia, thereby increasing insulin requirements. However, for high protein–low carbohydrate meals (e.g., steak and salad), at least 75 g of protein (equivalent to ~8 oz steak) is needed before a significant effect is seen. Indeed, 75 g of protein alone has been shown to increase blood glucose levels to the same extent as 20 g of carbohydrate without insulin. As with dietary fat, the effects of protein are delayed and typically are seen ~1.5 h after the meal.

Meals high in fat and protein require more insulin to control late-postprandial hyperglycemia than low-fat, low-protein meals with the same carbohydrate content, the actual amount of additional insulin and the insulin delivery pattern required for high-fat or high-protein meals is not clear. Preliminary studies have indicated that for individuals using insulin pump therapy, a combo, extended, or dual-wave bolus extending over 2–2.5 h with as much as a 35% increased meal bolus may be necessary. Alternatively, patients using MDI may need to cover the meal with a preprandial injection of regular insulin with or without analog insulin. In practice, it would be advisable to start with dose increases of 15–20% for high-protein and 30–35% of high-fat meals, accompanied with close monitoring and frequent reviews. Doses can be titrated as needed.

WEIGHT GAIN ASSOCIATED WITH INTENSIVE MANAGEMENT

Weight gain may accompany intensive management as tighter blood glucose control is achieved, and it affects patients regardless of age or sex. Factors thought to be associated with weight gain are failure to compensate for calories no longer lost via glycosuria, consumption of extra calories to treat more frequent episodes of hypoglycemia, or repletion of body water or protein lost during a period of poor glucose control. In addition, patients on intensive therapy may find that they can consume a greater variety of foods without loss of glucose control and, therefore, experience the same result from overeating as the rest of the population.

PREVENTION

Experience suggests that the following strategies may be helpful (see Table 9.8):

- **Reduce caloric intake at the initiation of intensive management.** A detailed nutrition history should be used to negotiate a meal plan that is 250–500 kcal less than that consumed before intensification of therapy, depending on degree of control before undertaking intensive management. The rationale for this change should be explained carefully.
- **Eliminate between-meal snacks.** For many patients, traditional between-meal snacks necessitated by insulin regimens that include intermediate-acting or regular insulin are one of the inconveniences of diabetes management. Many patients are willing to eliminate snacks as a means to reduce caloric intake. A consistent need for snacks between meals to avoid hypoglycemia may indicate that the basal insulin dose is excessive. Children and adolescents may need snacks to provide appropriate calories for normal

growth. Many young children have a snack in the middle of the morning and in the afternoon, and may eat again before going to bed. Older children and adolescents generally have an afterschool snack and may or may not have a snack before bed.

■ **Treat hypoglycemia with glucose.** Treating hypoglycemia with foods that contain fat or protein in addition to carbohydrate slows the correction of hypoglycemia and leads to increased caloric intake. Therefore, patients should be urged to avoid treating hypoglycemia with common snack foods such as cheese and crackers or candy bars. The appropriate amount of carbohydrate, preferably in the form of glucose (see the section Oral Treatment of Hypoglycemia) should be consumed to correct hypoglycemia.

■ **Initiate an exercise program as part of intensive management.** The type and amount of exercise should be individualized. Current exercise recommendations for most adults are to aim for at least 30 min of moderate-intensity activity on most, if not all, days of the week, or ~150 min of exercise per week. The exercise program should also include resistance exercise, in addition to aerobic exercise, which can improve insulin sensitivity in people with T2D.

■ **Decrease insulin doses for activity that exceeds daily routines.** Traditional dogma has taught patients to eat more when they exercise more than usual, a practice that makes weight control more difficult. With practice and judicious use of blood glucose monitoring, patients can become skilled at reducing their usual insulin doses to offset the effect of additional exercise.

Table 9.8—Prevention of Weight Gain During Intensive Management

- Reduce calore intake by 250–500 kcal/day
- Eliminate between-meal snacks
- Treat hypoglycemia with measured amounts of glucose
- Initiate or increase physical activity
- Decrease insulin for exercise instead of snacking

BIBLIOGRAPHY

American Diabetes Association. *ADA Guide to Nutrition Therapy for Diabetes* 2nd Edition. Alexandria, VA, American Diabetes Association, 2012.

American Diabetes Association/Academy of Nutrition and Dietetics. *Count Your Carbs: Getting Started.* Alexandria, VA, American Diabetes Association; Chicago, Academy of Nutrition and Dietetics, 2014

American Diabetes Association/Academy of Nutrition and Dietetics. *Match Your Insulin to Your Carbs.* Alexandria, VA, American Diabetes Association; Chicago, Academy of Nutrition and Dietetics, 2014

Bell KJ, Smart CE, Steil GM, Brand-Miller JC, King B, Wolpert HA. Impact of fat, protein, and glycemic index on postprandial glucose control in type 1 diabetes: implications for intensive diabetes management in the continuous glucose monitoring era. *Diabetes Care* 2015;38:1008–1015

Delahanty LM, Halford BN. The role of diet behaviors in achieving improved glycemic control in intensively treated patients in the Diabetes Control and Complications Trial. *Diabetes Care* 1993;16:1453–1458

Diabetes Control and Complications Trial (DCCT) Research Group. Weight gain associated with intensive therapy in the Diabetes Control and Complications Trial. *Diabetes Care* 1988;11:567–573

Diabetes Control and Complications Trial (DCCT) Research Group: Nutrition interventions for intensive therapy in the Diabetes Control and Complications Trial. *J Am Diet Assoc* 1993;93:768–772

Diabetes Control and Complications Trial (DCCT) Research Group. Expanded role of the dietitian in the Diabetes Control and Complications Trial: implications for clinical practice. *J Am Diet Assoc* 1994;93:758–767

Estruch R, Ros E, Salas-Salvado J, et al. Primary prevention of cardiovascular disease with a Mediterranean diet. *N Engl J Med* 2013;368:1279–1290

Evert A, Boucher J, Cypress M, et al. American Diabetes Association position statement: nutrition therapy recommendations for the management of adults with diabetes. *Diabetes Care* 2013;36:3821–3842

Franz MJ, Boucher JL, Green-Pastors J, Power MA. Evidence-based nutrition practice guidelines for diabetes and scope and standards of practice. *J Am Diet Assoc* 2008;108(Suppl.):S52–S58

Garg S, Zisser H, Schwartz S, Bailey T, Kaplan R, Ellis S, Jovanovic L. Improvement in glycemic excursions with a transcutaneous, real-time continuous glucose sensor: a randomized control trial. *Diabetes Care* 2006;29:44–50

Juvenile Diabetes Research Foundation Continuous Glucose Monitoring Study Group; Tamborlane WV, Beck RW, Bode BW, Buckingham B, Chase HP, Clemons R, Fiallo-Scharer R, Fox LA, Gilliam LK, Hirsch IB, Huang ES, Kollman C, Kowalski AJ, Laffel L, Lawrence JM, Lee J, Mauras N, O'Grady M, Ruedy KJ, Tansey M, Tsalikian E, Weinzimer S, Wilson DM, Wolpert H, Wysocki T, Xing D. Continuous glucose monitoring and intensive treatment of type 1 diabetes. *N Engl J Med* 2008;359:1464–1476

Look AHEAD Research Group; PI-Sunyer X, Blackburn G, Brancati FL, et al. Long-term effects of a lifestyle intervention on weight and cardiovascular risk factors in individuals with type 2 diabetes mellitus: four-year results of the Look AHEAD trial. *Arch Intern Med* 2010;170:1566–1575

Warshaw H, Bolderman K. *Practical Carbohydrate Counting: A How-to-Teach Guide for Health Professionals*. 2nd ed. Alexandria, VA, American Diabetes Association, 2001

Index

Note: Page numbers followed by an *f* refer to figures. Page numbers followed by a *t* refer to tables.

I

iatrogenic hypoglycemia, 7
illness, 87, 98, 103, 121, 144
information, 26–27
informational support, 52
injection device, 89–90
injection port, 90
instruction, 28–29, 31–32
insulin
  absorption, 80–81, 103
  action, 6, 76–77
  adjustment, 87–89, 140, 148–149
  analog, 3
  aspart, 76, 77*t*, 78–80
  aspart protamine suspension (NPA),
    78–79
  basal, 7, 32*t*, 78–79, 81–85, 87, 89*t*,
    96–100, 103
  basal-bolus regimen, 85*f*, 130, 139
  bolus, 32*t*, 96–97, 100–101
  combination, 77*t*
  comparative action, 77*t*
  concentrated formulation, 79
  correction dose, 88
  degludec, 77*t*, 79–80, 83
  detemir, 77*t*, 78–80, 83–84, 143
  distribution, 86–87
  dose, 32*t*, 43, 86–87, 102, 148
  effect, 83*f*–86*f*
  exercise, 150
  fuel metabolism regulation, 6–7
  glargine, 77*t*, 79–80, 83, 143
  glulisine, 76, 77*t*, 79–80
  injection site, 80
  intermediate-acting, 77–78, 82, 84,
    85*f*, 142–143
  lispro, 76, 77*t*, 78–80
  lispro protamine suspension (NPL),
    78–79
  long-acting, 77*t*, 78, 82–83
  meal,inappropriate timing relative to,
    143–144
  mixture, 78–79
  multicomponent regimen, 76–90
  NPH, 77–79

  nutrition assessment, 134*t*
  pattern adjustment, 87, 89
  pen, 79, 90
  pharmacology, 76–81
  prandial, 7, 81–82, 87, 136–137
  premeal basal intermediate-acting,
    84–85
  premeal injection timing, 80–81
  premeal rapid-acting, 83–84
  preprandial, 82–83
  profile, 82*f*
  rapid-acting, 76–77, 79–83, 84*f*, 85–86,
    88, 89*t*, 98, 101, 136, 143
  regimen, 81–86
  regular, 77*t*, 78–81
  restriction, 44–46
  secretion, 7–8, 81
  sensitivity, 5, 85, 140
  short-acting, 77, 77*t*, 84*f*–85*f*, 142–143
  sliding scale, 88
  stability, 79–80
  storage, 79
  subcutaneous injection site, 8
  timing, 76
  type 1 diabetes (T1D), 136
  type 2 diabetes (T2D), 5
  U-100 glargine, 78, 83
  ultralong-acting, 77*t*, 78–79, 82
insulin-induced hypoglycemia, 145
insulin infusion pump therapy, 96–110
  dosage calculation, 98–101
  glucose control, erratic, 111*t*
  hypoglycemia, fear of, 43–44
  infusion set, 103
  intensive diabetes management
    success, 3–4
  ketone monitoring, 121
  meal bolus, 149
  multicomponent regimen, 86
  patient education, 107*t*, 109–110
  patient selection criteria, 99*t*
  pump, wearing the, 108–109
  risks of, 103–108
  technical components, 110*t*
insulin on board, 98

medical nutrition therapy, 130
microvascular complication, 47
multicomponent regimen, 81
nutrition, 134*t*, 136–137
real-time continuous glucose
    monitoring (RT-CGM), 111
retinal examination, 124
self-controlled coping, 48
studies, 3
total daily dose (TDD), 99
urinary albumin screening, 125
type 2 diabetes (T2D), 130
    acute insulin adjustment, 88
    binge eating, 45–46
    blood glucose monitoring, 141*t*
    intensive diabetes management, 40
    intensive management strategies, 4
    lifestyle change, 50
    macrovascular complication, 47
    nutrition, 134*t*, 137–139
    patients, 65–67
    psychological insulin resistance, 44
    retinal examination, 124
    studies, 3
    total daily dose (TDD), 99

U

UK Prospective Diabetes Study
    (UKPDS), 3, 47, 50
urinary albumin screening, 123*t*, 125
urine ketone testing, 120–121
urine-monitoring strip, 120
USDA Choose My Plate Guidelines;
    Dietary Guidelines for Americans,
    147*t*

V

very low-calorie diets (VLCDs), 138
Veterans Affairs Diabetes Trial [VADT],
    3
vomiting, 45

W

weight, 44–45, 65–66, 137–139, 149–150